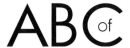
ABC of

One to Seven

Fifth Edition

EDITED BY

Bernard Valman
Consultant Paediatrician
Northwick Park Hospital, London, UK
Honorary Senior Lecturer
Imperial College London, UK

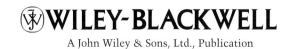
WILEY-BLACKWELL
A John Wiley & Sons, Ltd., Publication

BMJ|Books

Library of Congress Cataloging-in-Publication Data
ABC of one to seven / edited by Bernard Valman; with contributions from Arlene Baroda ... [et al.]. -- 5th ed.
    p. ; cm.
    Includes bibliographical references and index.
    ISBN 978-1-4051-8105-1
    1. Pediatrics--Handbooks, manuals, etc. I. Valman, H. B. (Hyman Bernard) II. Baroda, Arlene.
    [DNLM: 1. Pediatrics. 2. Child Development. 3. Child Health Services. WS 100 A134 2009]
    RJ48.A23 2009
    618.92--dc22

                                                                                          2009004428

ISBN: 978-1-4051-8105-1

A catalogue record for this book is available from the British Library.

Set in 9.25/12 pt Minion by Newgen Imaging Systems (P) Ltd, Chennai, India
Printed and bound in Singapore by Ho Printing Singapore Pte Ltd

1   2010

Contents

Contributors, vii

Preface, viii

1 Talking to Children, 1
Bernard Valman

2 The Terrible Twos, 3
Claire Sturge

3 Sleep Problems, 6
Bernard Valman

4 Respiratory Tract Infection, 10
Bernard Valman

5 Tonsillitis and Otitis Media, 14
Bernard Valman

6 Stridor, 18
Bernard Valman

7 Asthma, 21
Bernard Valman

8 Acute Abdominal Pain, 28
Bernard Valman

9 Recurrent Abdominal Pain, 32
Bernard Valman

10 Vomiting and Acute Diarrhoea, 35
Bernard Valman

11 Chronic Diarrhoea, 39
Bernard Valman

12 Urinary Tract Infection, 43
Bernard Valman

13 Nocturnal Enuresis, 48
Bernard Valman

14 Systolic Murmurs, 51
Bernard Valman

15 Growth Failure, 53
Bernard Valman

16 Prevention and Management of Obesity, 57
Bernard Valman

17 Common Rashes, 60
Bernard Valman

18 Infectious Diseases, 64
Bernard Valman

19 Paediatric Dermatology, 69
Saleem Goolamali

20 Febrile Convulsions, 77
Bernard Valman

21 Epilepsy, 80
Bernard Valman

22 Recurrent Headache, 83
Bernard Valman

23 Poisoning, 86
Bernard Valman

24 Accidents, 90
Bernard Valman

25 Severely Ill Children, 94
Bernard Valman

26 Basic Life Support in the Community, 100
Bernard Valman

27 The Child with Fever, 102
Bernard Valman

28 Behaviour Problems, 105
Bernard Valman

29 Children with Special Needs, 108
Daphne Keen

30 School Failure, 112
Ruth Levere

31 Minor Orthopaedic Problems, 115
John Fixsen

32 Limp, 119
John Fixsen

33 Services for Children: Primary Care, 122
Ed Peile

34 Services for Children: The Community, 128
Arlene Boroda

35 Services for Children: Outpatient Clinics and Day-Care, 131
Bernard Valman

36 Services for Children: Emergency Department, Ambulatory, and Inpatients, 134
Bernard Valman

37 Audit in Primary Care Paediatrics, 138
Ed Peile

38 Child Abuse, 141
Arlene Boroda

39 Services for Children: Children's Social Care, 144
Ron Lock

40 Useful Information, 147
Bernard Valman

Acknowledgements, 153

Index, 154

Contributors

Arlene Boroda

North West London NHS Trust, London, UK

John Fixsen

Emeritus Consultant Orthopaedic Surgeon, Great
Ormond Street Children's Hospital, London, UK

Saleem Goolamali

Consultant Dermatologist, Clementine Churchill Hospital, Harrow, UK

Daphne Keen

Consultant Developmental Paediatrician, St George's Hospital, London, UK

Ruth Levere

Consultant Clinical Psychologist, Child and
Adolescent Mental Health Services, Harrow, UK

Ron Lock

Independent Child Protection Consultant, Salisbury, UK

Ed Peile

Professor of Medical Education, University of Warwick, Coventry, UK

Claire Sturge

Consultant Child Psychiatrist, Child and Adolescent
Mental Health Services, Harrow, UK

Bernard Valman

Consultant Paediatrician, Northwick Park Hospital, London, UK,
and Honorary Senior Lecturer, Imperial College London, UK

Preface

Practice rather than theory is the keynote of *ABC of One to Seven* in its straightforward advice on the diseases, emotional problems, and developmental disorders of early childhood. Considerable changes have been made in this edition to bring every page up to date. The format has been enhanced to make the material more attractive to the reader and all the illustrations are now in colour. New chapters include the prevention and management of obesity, behavioural and emotional problems, the child with fever, and basic life support. Several chapters have been completely rewritten by new authors and reflect the extensive changes in management since the last edition. These chapters include children with special needs, school failure, child abuse, services for children in the community, primary care, audit in primary care, and children's social services. The management of problems which are being recognized more frequently such as attention deficit hyperactivity disorder (ADHD) have been covered more extensively in this edition. As each chapter has been designed for the management of a specific clinical feature, overlap has been inevitable but the advice is consistent.

The latest clinical guidelines from NICE (National Institute for Health and Clinical Excellence) have been incorporated in the text and relevant websites and publications are given at the end of each chapter. Authoritative websites that can be accessed during a consultation with a patient are found in the chapter on primary care.

The *ABC of One to Seven* and the companion book, *ABC of the First Year*, have become standard guides for general practitioners, doctors in the training grades both in the community and hospital, medical students, midwives, nurses, and health visitors. They have become indispensable reference books for GP surgeries, emergency and outpatient departments, wards, and libraries.

For ease of reading and simplicity a single pronoun has been used for feminine and masculine subjects; a specific gender is not implied.

Bernard Valman

CHAPTER 1

Talking to Children

Bernard Valman

Northwick Park Hospital and Imperial College London, UK

OVERVIEW

- The newborn share with lovers the ability to speak with the eyes. Communication develops from unintelligible sounds to gestures and finally words. An adult elicits these responses from a healthy child by normal speech or appropriate books or toys (Figure 1.1).

- Failure to respond may provide important evidence that there is a delay in development or a defect in the special senses. A quick response may help to distinguish between a child with a trivial problem who is just tired and a child with a severe illness such as septicaemia.

- Although guidelines on approaching children can be given, a normal range can be learnt only by attempting to communicate with every child.

In the consulting room

While the history is being taken from the parent the child will be listening and watching even if he appears preoccupied with play. If the doctor has formed a good rapport with the parent the child may talk easily when approached.

A small table and chair are needed at one side of the doctor's desk, and toys suitable for each age group should be scattered on this table, on the floor, and on adjacent shelves (Figure 1.2). The normal toddler will usually rush to this table and play. He remains quiet and while the history is being taken the doctor can observe the child's development of play, temperament, and dependence on his parents and the relationship between the parents and child. When the child is playing happily the doctor can wander over and start a conversation about the toys he has chosen. Even if the doctor knows a great deal about levels of communication and development the mother will display the child's abilities by talking to him herself. By observing her first, the doctor can pitch the method and type of communication at the right level. Ideally, the eyes of the child and the doctor should be on the same horizontal plane so the doctor may have to sit on the floor, kneel, or crouch. Adequate time should be given to allow the child to respond, particularly those who cannot say words.

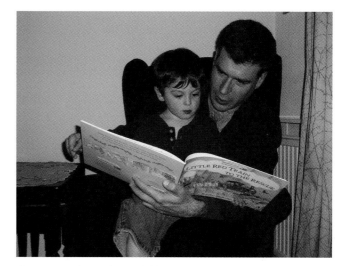
Figure 1.1 Father reading to child.

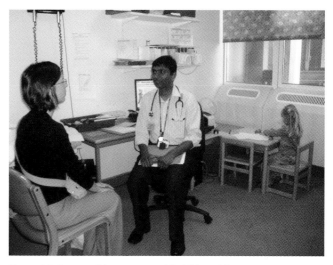
Figure 1.2 Doctor talking to parent with child at table.

Questioning the child

An older child should be encouraged to sit nearest to the doctor and it may be possible to prompt him to give the history (Figure 1.3). A history taken directly from the child is often the most accurate, although the parent may need to supply the duration and frequency

ABC of One to Seven, 5th edition. Edited by B. Valman. © 2010 Blackwell Publishing, ISBN: 978-1-4051-8105-1.

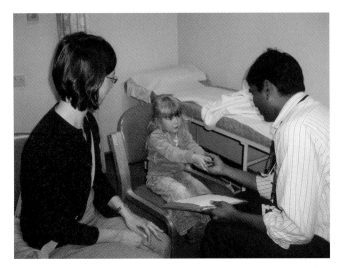

Figure 1.3 Doctor talking to child with parent.

of the symptoms. The first words determine the success of the interview. The question 'Where is the site of your abdominal pain, John?' will be greeted by silence. Questions that might start the conversation include 'Which television programme do you like best?' 'Did you come to the surgery by bus or car?' 'What did you have for breakfast?' It may be necessary to make it clear to the mother that the doctor wants to hear what the child has to say. She may interpose answers because she may think that she can give a more accurate history, wants to avert criticism, is overprotective, or wants to save the doctor's time. Ideally, the child and the parents should be seen together and later separately, but children who do not speak freely in the presence of their parents are unlikely, during the first visit, to speak more openly when they are separated.

The child should be addressed by his own name or the nickname that he likes. A little flattery sometimes helps, for example, admiring a girl's dress or saying that a toddler is grown up. A cheeky smile in response to a question as to whether a boy fights with his sister shows that you are on the right wavelength. For children who are not yet talking it may be possible to play a simple game of putting things into a cup and taking them out or making scribbles on a piece of paper alternately with the child. Simple words should be used which the child is likely to understand, but if a doctor uses a childish word when the patient knows it by a normal word he will think that the doctor is treating him as a baby and underestimating his abilities.

Reassuring parents and children

Before starting a physical examination say to the child 'Is it alright for me to examine you now, just as your own doctor does?' The child's reaction will give an indication whether there will be resistance to an examination and whether only partial examination will be possible at that visit. It gives formal consent and shows that the child is an individual with personal rights.

Whatever the age, talking to a child during an examination has several advantages. If the doctor says, 'That's good' after listening to the heart for a long time this reassures the mother that nothing dreadful has been found. Saying to the child, 'You are very good this time' or 'You are very grown up' often keeps the child still while his ears are being examined or abdomen palpated. Even if the child does not understand the meaning of the words, the tone of the examiner's voice may calm him and allow prolonged detailed examination without protest.

Going to the doctor should be a treat, so more exciting books, toys, and equipment should be available than are present at home. In the past many doctors used sweets to soften the trauma of a visit to the surgery but many parents now frown on doctors who have apparently not heard the advice of dentists. A sweet in the mouth of the child during examination of the throat can be dangerous. A properly equipped waiting room and consulting room provide an incentive for the child to come again.

Further reading

Byron T. *Your Toddler Month by Month*. Dorling Kindersley, London, 2008.

CHAPTER 2

The Terrible Twos

Claire Sturge

Child and Adolescent Mental Health Services, Harrow, UK

> **OVERVIEW**
>
> - The period between 2 and 3 years of age may bring disillusion to parents. Their idealised innocent angel seems to have become a calculating tyrant.
> - Until then the words 'mischievous', 'naughty', 'little devil' were terms of endearment. At 2 years they become accurate terms of description: the child's behaviour appears to be planned to cause the maximum anguish.
> - Understanding the reasons for the behaviour and providing firm, consistent responses produces a change in the child's behaviour and a reduction in the parents' feelings of inadequacy.

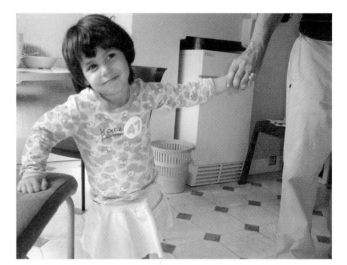

Figure 2.1 Showing independence by pulling away from father.

Independence versus dependence

At about the age of 2 years children discover that they can control what happens around them when they begin to talk and can decide when to pass urine or stools. A conflict develops between their desire to assert their independence (Figure 2.1) and their wish to regress to an earlier stage of dependence. The independence may be expressed in the defiance of temper tantrums, but increasing independence can bring anxiety and a sense of insecurity. This can lead to clinginess, separation anxiety, fears and phobias or security seeking behaviours such as continual use of a blanket or other transitional object. The conflict between seeking independence and seeking the security of dependence is seen in lapses in sphincter control, awkward behaviour in relation to eating and brief periods of speech regression.

At the age of 2 years symbolic thought is just beginning to develop, but it is self-centred. This newly developed level of understanding and command of speech combined with a disregard for the needs of others may lead the parents to think that their child is determined to thwart or hurt them. A mother might be trying to dress a 2-year-old quickly to be on time for an appointment, but he treats the whole event as a game, running and hiding, and does not understand why his mother loses her temper. These episodes also illustrate the toddler's inability to see any behaviour from the other person's point of view. A violent temper tantrum, even when he kicks or bites his mother, is not about hurting his mother but about trying to assert control.

At this age there is also little sense of time so the child does not understand urgency or the need to hurry up or wait. A few minutes of separation from his mother may seem like for ever and the child's response to such separations will depend on their pattern of attachment – secure (is confident enough about his carer's ability to manage his distress to manage a short separation without reacting angrily or dismissively) or insecure (is unsure about his mother's reliability and shows avoidance or anxiety even when reunited). Mishandling separations can have long-term sequelae: telling your child you are just popping to the toilet when actually you are leaving the house or playgroup undermines the child's trust in you.

Effects on parents

The other half of the picture of the terrible 2-year-old is the distraught parents, particularly the mother. Mothers often feel that they cannot cope and become depressed and anxious. Their families, friends, and husbands may support them, but being socially isolated or disadvantaged can have an adverse effect on parenting capacity. The referral rate for 2- to 3-year-olds to family doctors is the highest of any age group, including the elderly.

ABC of One to Seven, 5th edition. Edited by B. Valman. © 2010 Blackwell Publishing, ISBN: 978-1-4051-8105-1.

The consultations are usually ostensibly about coughs and colds, but the real reason may be that the mother is having great difficulty in coping with her toddler. The problems are best seen as interactional (i.e. as in the dynamic relationship between child and carer not located simply in one or the other). An accurate formulation of the dyadic (mother–child) problems and sound advice at this stage can be an important part of preventive child health.

Two years is also a common age gap between children, so the mother may be pregnant or just have had another baby. The toddler may show resentment, sometimes very intense, towards the new baby, and the parents feel hurt by this resentment. Complex expressions of this resentment (e.g. the toddler who half suffocates the new baby with embraces may deceive parents into believing the new addition is adored). Misunderstanding the young child's feelings can reinforce the confusion of feelings in the 2-year-old and worsen or may precipitate behaviour seen in this age group, and may lead to parents questioning where they went wrong in bringing up their child. Parents need to see this as a necessary and healthy developmental stage which they need to work through with their child.

Intervention

Every baby is born with a different temperament. This is innate and largely genetically determined and there is nothing the parents can do to change this endowment. Children vary in their moodiness, response to frustration, intensity of responses, and adaptability (Figure 2.2). They also vary in the intervals between micturition and defecation, the regularity of their bodily functions, and their need for sleep and food. The 'easiest' child temperamentally is a child who is not very intense or moody, has a high threshold for frustration, is not particularly active, and adapts easily. Such a child may not present any particular problems at 2. The converse

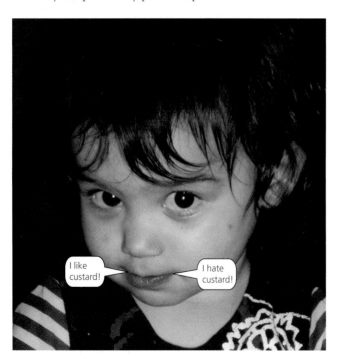

Figure 2.2 Mood changes quickly.

describes a 'difficult' child. If this variability is explained to the parents it may improve their understanding of their child, remove some of their guilt, and enable them to handle the child better. It is well established that 'sensitive parenting' is the key to children's healthy emotional development.

Intervention is effective only if the parents can see the child's problem in perspective and are more concerned with resolving it than with concentrating on the feelings the child's behaviour arouses in them. Many of the problems 2-year-olds pose are habit problems – for example, sleep problems – and the habits have developed because the parents have reinforced them in some way. Despite the parents' bitter complaints about their child's behaviour they are often unable to change their own behaviour. For example, if a 2-year-old's frequent temper tantrums make his mother feel that she is responsible for his unhappiness and she thinks that the tantrums are a sign of insecurity, she will not be firm with the child and will not follow the doctor's advice. Such firmness actually reassures the child and makes the child feel more secure – someone takes control when he cannot.

Families often claim to have tried everything when in fact they have not pursued one specific method with commitment. They may see any intervention as cruel and unloving. If the mother realises that she, the child, and the family would have an easier time if there were fewer tantrums she can be advised to ignore them. She must ignore them every time and, if necessary, leave the child alone in the room or put him in another one. When the child is finally calm, however long this takes, she should then behave normally and accept the child fully; she should never give additional treats in the form of sweets or cuddles.

Behavioural studies show that if children find that they can ever 'get away' with a particular form of behaviour they will repeatedly try it out because they know that exceptions to the new, firm response are possible. The parents need to know that any inconsistency will lead to failure: inconsistency in discipline reinforces the behaviour the parent is trying to eliminate. When the child realises that both parents have an agreed and consistent approach the temper tantrums will stop.

Sleeping, eating, and continence

The approach to sleeping problems is similar to that for temper tantrums and requires a behavioural approach aimed at instilling bedtime routines and the child learning to settle himself to sleep. Graded approaches are usually successful, such as getting the child to sleep at an increasing distance from his parent or spending progressively less time in the child's room settling him to sleep. Bright lights near the child in the hour before sleep (e.g. TV), suppresses the 'sleep hormone' melatonin and should be avoided.

Healthy toddlers gain weight normally in spite of their mother's anxieties about their poor eating or being very fussy. Children know their minimum requirements instinctively. Refusal to eat is a very powerful weapon as it is experienced by the mother as a challenge to her maternal ability to nurture her child. If the mother is reassured that the child will not harm himself by not eating, then conflicts which at this age tend to reinforce the behaviour, can be avoided.

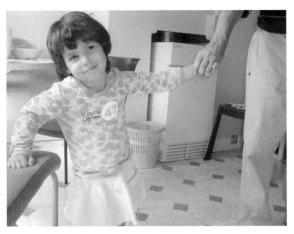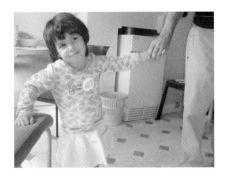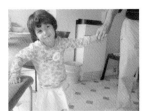

Figure 2.3 Problems appear smaller by 3 years.

Toilet training may be tackled either by highly structured training schemes or by waiting and reattempting training at intervals. Problems around continence are common as this is another area where the child is testing out his newfound areas of control. Many 2-year-old children have problems with bladder and bowel control at some time, but in most they resolve spontaneously at the age of 3 or 4.

Problems of dependence

Problems relating to dependence, such as fears and phobias, excessive use of security items, excessive masturbation, or nightmares, need a very different approach and it is the parents who need most help in understanding the problems and helping the child. They need to learn not to reinforce the anxieties by overreacting to the child's fear or behaviour, but to help the child learn to feel in control of his situation and more confident. Encouraging children to play or act out things they worry about may help. Separation fears are a common anxiety, even when there seems no real reason for them.

Difficulty in separation at this age is normal and should not be seen as a problem. Giving 2-year-olds a positive experience of separation will increase their resilience – learning they can trust their mother to return will make them more confident and less vulnerable. This is a good age for introducing such experiences with people they know well if such experiences are not already established.

Better by three

As children approach the age of 3 years they become more sociable and learn to share and to take turns. They are also more proficient at communicating. Most will have mastered control of their bladder and bowel, and other control issues slowly become less problematic over the next year or two.

All the problems discussed here are variations in behaviour that fall within the normal range. When doctors are consulted they may find themselves unable to help because the family does not genuinely want to change the way it behaves or go through the process of altering their parenting practices, in which case reassurance that the child's behaviour will probably improve with time may be all that can be done (Figure 2.3).

Whether or not the family is receptive or resistant to advice, an explanation of why the child behaves as he does may be valuable and help to make the parents feel understood. The doctor or health visitor is in a good position to advise on toddler management and many advice sheets are available (as well as advice on the Internet). If the child's behaviour or the family's reaction to it is well outside the normal range then he should be referred to a children's centre, parent training programme, or child mental health service. If the whole family is disrupted by the child's behaviour, particularly where there is risk that the stress to the parent might result in some harm to the child, a referral to Children's Social Care may be needed.

Underlying problems that may contribute to or explain behaviour problems must always be considered and those with developmental problems such as persisting language, hearing, or speech problems, features suggestive of global (e.g. a learning disability) or pervasive developmental delay (e.g. indicators of autism), should be referred to a specialist service.

Further reading

Byron T. *Your Toddler Month by Month*. Dorling Kindersley, London, 2008.
Prior V, Glaser D. *Understanding Attachment and Attachment Disorders: Theory, Evidence and Practice*. Child and Adolescent Mental Health Series. The Royal College of Psychiatrists. Atheneum Press, Gateshead, 2006.

CHAPTER 3

Sleep Problems

Bernard Valman

Northwick Park Hospital and Imperial College London, UK

OVERVIEW

- Some children will not sleep when they are put to bed, but the most distressing problem for parents is those who keep waking in the night or wake in the early morning. The parents rapidly become exhausted, and parental discord may follow, while the child remains fresh.

- Sleep problems are common. Twenty per cent of infants wake early or in the night at the age of 2, and it is still a problem in 10% at 4½. Between these ages the symptoms resolve in some children but appear for the first time in others.

- Bedtime rituals may prevent sleep problems and simple behaviour modification methods may reduce them.

- Drugs, for example salbutamol given for asthma, may cause irritability and sleep problems.

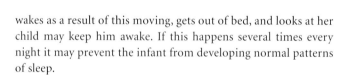

Figure 3.1 Large range in normal sleep patterns.

Normal patterns

During the first few weeks of life some babies sleep almost continuously for the 24 hours whereas others sleep for only about 12 hours (Figure 3.1). This pattern of needing little sleep may persist so that by the age of 1 year an infant may wake regularly at 02.00 hours and remain awake for 2 hours or more. As these infants approach the age of 3 they tend to wake at 06.00 hours and then remain awake for the rest of the day. Many 2-year-old children sleep for an hour or two in the afternoons, and some have a similar amount of sleep in the mornings as well. A child who spends 4 hours of the day sleeping may spend 4 hours of the night awake. Parents often worry that an infant is suffering from lack of sleep and wrongly ascribe poor appetite or frequent colds to this cause.

During the night babies and children often wake up, open their eyes, lift their heads, and move their limbs. If they are not touched most of them fall back to sleep again. A mother who wakes as a result of this moving, gets out of bed, and looks at her child may keep him awake. If this happens several times every night it may prevent the infant from developing normal patterns of sleep.

History

A full history should be taken. Essential details are the sleep pattern, when the problem began, and measures taken to resolve it. It should be possible to determine whether the child has always needed little sleep or whether he has developed a habit of crying in order to get into his parents' comfortable bed. Doctors should also explore the reason why the mother has sought advice at this stage. She should be asked about any change in the house, where the child sleeps, whether he attends a playgroup, and who looks after him during the day. Illnesses in the child or family and parental and social backgrounds should be considered.

Nightmares may occur after any trauma such as a frightening programme on television or bullying at school. Night terrors

ABC of One to Seven, 5th edition. Edited by B. Valman. © 2010 Blackwell Publishing, ISBN: 978-1-4051-8105-1.

are a rare form of nightmare in which the child wakes at exactly the same time every night. He may appear not to recognise his parents and is not consoled by them. Waking him half an hour before the expected episode each night for a week alters the sleep pattern and may resolve the symptoms.

A physical examination usually shows no abnormality, but occasionally there may be signs of acute otitis media.

Difficulty in going to sleep

Difficulty in getting to sleep can often be avoided by starting a bedtime ritual in infancy. A warm bath followed by being wrapped in particular blankets may later be replaced by the mother or father reading from a book or singing nursery rhymes before the light is turned out (Figure 3.2). Some children have been frightened by a nightmare and fear going to sleep in case it is repeated. A small night light or a light on the landing showing through the open door may allay this fear. A soft cuddly toy of any type can lie next to the infant from shortly after birth, and seeing this familiar toy again may help to induce sleep.

The mother should be told that during the night babies often open their eyes and move their limbs and heads. She should be asked to resist getting up to see the baby as the noise of getting out of bed may wake him and he may then remain awake. If he does wake he may be pacified with a drink and may then fall asleep. The drink is to provide comfort rather than to reduce any thirst.

Parents whose young children sleep a great deal during the day can discourage them from doing this by taking them out shopping or giving them other diversions and they may then sleep well at night.

Sleep disturbance is a common reaction to the trauma of admission to hospital or moving house. Taking the child into the parents' room, to sleep in his own cot or bed, for a few weeks

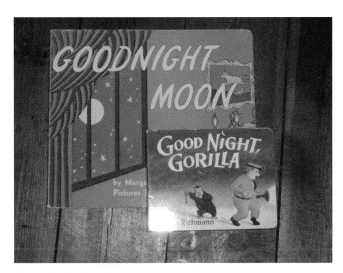

Figure 3.2 Bedtime story book.

may help to reassure the child that he has not been abandoned. If there are toys or other things to amuse them some children who wake in the night will play for hours, talking to themselves and not crying. Parents need to be reassured that this is perfectly normal and that they are lucky that the child does not demand their attention.

If the child is prepared to go to sleep at a certain time but the parents would like to advance it by an hour they can put him to bed 5 minutes earlier each night until the planned bedtime is achieved.

Behaviour modification and drugs

When children wake frequently during the night and cry persistently until they are taken into the parents' bed a plan of action is needed. If there is an obvious cause, such as acute illness, recent admission to hospital, or a new baby, the problem may resolve itself within a few weeks, and at first there need be no change in management. If there is no obvious cause the parents are asked to keep a record of the child's sleep pattern and their action when the child woke for 2 weeks (Boxes 3.1 and 3.2). This helps to determine where the main problem lies and can be used as a comparison with treatment.

Both parents are seen at the next visit; both need to accept that they must be firm and follow the plan exactly. Behaviour modification is the only method that produces long-term improvement, but it can be combined with drugs initially if the mother is at breaking point.

Behaviour modification separates the mother from the child gradually or abruptly, depending on the parents' and doctor's philosophy. The slow method starts with the mother giving a drink and staying with the child for decreasing lengths of time. In the next stage no drink is given. Then she speaks to the child through the closed door and, finally, does not go to him at all. The abrupt method consists of letting the child cry it out; he stops after three or four nights. There are infinite numbers of variations between these extremes, and the temperament of the parents, child, and doctor will determine what is acceptable.

Another approach is to increase the waiting time before going to the child (Table 3.1). In severe cases a written programme of several small changes can be given to the mother and she can be seen again by the health visitor or family doctor after each step has been achieved. The mother will need to be reassured and neighbours may be pacified by being told that the child will soon be cured.

Many sleep problems can be resolved without drugs, but some mothers are so exhausted by loss of sleep that they cannot manage a programme of behaviour modification unless the infant receives some preliminary sedation. The most satisfactory drug in this age group is chloral hydrate 30 mg/kg body weight given 1 hour before going to bed. The full dose is given for 1 week, followed by a half dose for a week; the drug is then given on alternate nights for a week. The objective is to change the pattern of sleeping. A behaviour modification plan is needed during the second and subsequent weeks.

Box 3.1 **Sleep history**

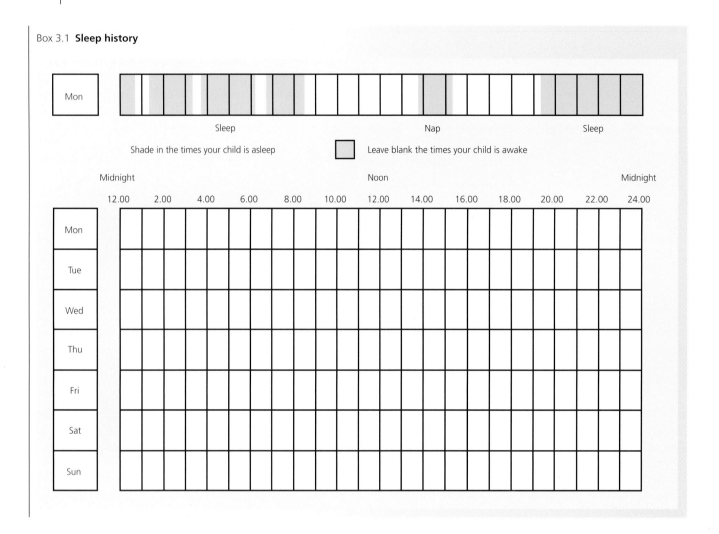

Box 3.2 **Parents' response**

Day	Time to bed	Time sleep	First problem	What did you do?	Second problem	What did you do?	Time woke up in the morning
Mon							
Tue							
Wed							
Thu							
Fri							
Sat							
Sun							

Table 3.1 Number of minutes to wait before going to your child briefly.

Day	At first episode	If your child is still crying		
		Second episode	Third episode	Subsequent episodes
1	5	10	15	15
2	10	15	20	20
3	15	20	25	25
4	20	25	30	30
5	25	30	35	35

Children around the age of 2 who wake early in the morning may be helped by giving them a low divan bed instead of a cot. They can get out of bed and play with their toys on the floor without disturbing others (Figure 3.3).

Further reading

Byron T. *Your Toddler Month by Month.* Dorling Kindersley, London, 2008.

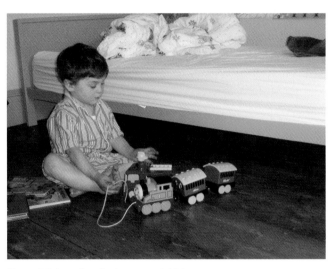

Figure 3.3 Low divan bed – toys and child.

CHAPTER 4

Respiratory Tract Infection

Bernard Valman

Northwick Park Hospital and Imperial College London, UK

> **OVERVIEW**
>
> - Although pathogens are often not confined to anatomical boundaries, respiratory tract infections may be classified as: (a) upper respiratory tract – common cold, tonsillitis and pharyngitis, and acute otitis media; (b) middle respiratory tract – acute laryngitis and epiglottitis; (c) lower respiratory tract – bronchitis, bronchopneumonia, and segmental pneumonia.
> - Viruses, which cause most respiratory tract infections, and bacterial infections produce similar clinical illnesses. Different viruses may produce an identical picture, or the same virus may cause different clinical syndromes. Clinically, it may not be possible to determine whether the infection is caused by viruses, bacteria, or both. If the infection is suspected of being bacterial, or the child has severe symptoms, it is safest to prescribe an antibiotic, as the results of virus studies are often received after the acute symptoms have passed.
> - The most common bacterial pathogens are pneumococci and *Haemophilus influenzae*. Less common are group A β haemolytic streptococci, *Staphylococcus aureus*, group B β haemolytic streptococci, Gram-negative bacteria, and anaerobic bacteria.

Common cold (coryza)

Preschool children usually have about six colds each year. The main symptoms are sneezing, nasal discharge, and mild fever. Similar symptoms may occur in the early phases of infection with rotavirus and be followed by vomiting and diarrhoea. Postnasal discharge may produce coughing. The most common complication is acute otitis media, but secondary bacterial infection of the lower respiratory tract sometimes occurs.

There is no specific treatment for the common cold, and antibiotics should not be given. It is helpful to explain to parents that antibiotics are not needed at that stage as they make no difference to the symptoms and may have side effects. Arrangements should be made for clinical review if the symptoms become worse or are prolonged beyond the following periods:

- Common cold 10 days
- Acute otitis media 4 days

ABC of One to Seven, 5th edition. Edited by B. Valman. © 2010 Blackwell Publishing, ISBN: 978-1-4051-8105-1.

- Acute sore throat 8 days
- Acute bronchitis or acute cough 3 weeks

A danger with nasal drops is that they will run down into the lower respiratory tract and carry the infection there. Recurrence of symptoms may occur if medicated nasal drops are used for more than 3 days.

Some children have severe symptoms every time they contract a viral infection, which is about once a month. If there are no signs of acute otitis media (see p. 14), paracetamol or ibuprofen to reduce the symptoms produced by fever is the only medication needed.

If the fever lasts less than 48 hours and the cough less than 3 weeks, no investigations are indicated and the parents can be reassured that the symptoms are likely to be less severe the following winter when immunity to common viruses will have improved.

Acute bronchitis

Acute bronchitis often follows a viral upper respiratory tract infection and there is always a cough, which may be accompanied by wheezing. There is no fever. The respiratory rate is normal (Table 4.1) and the symptoms resolve within 3 weeks. The only signs, which are not constantly present, are wheezes. As it is usually caused by a virus, antibiotics are indicated only if the illness is severe or a bacterial cause is shown. If there is no indication to give an antibiotic when the child is seen, the parents can be informed that an antibiotic is not needed at that time, as it would make no difference to the symptoms and may have side effects. Arrangements are made for clinical review if the symptoms become worse or are prolonged (see above). An alternative approach is to give this explanation and to

Table 4.1 Upper limit for normal respiratory and heart rate per minute at rest related to age.

Age	Respiratory rate	Heart rate
<2 months	60	160
2–11 months	40	160
12–24 months	35	150
2–5 years	30	140
5–12 years	25	120

give a prescription for an antibiotic, which can be given if specific criteria are satisfied. The child should be reviewed clinically if the symptoms become worse despite the antibiotic.

Recurrent bronchitis

Two separate episodes of acute bronchitis may occur in a normal child in a year. If attacks are more frequent at any age bronchial asthma should be considered (see p. 21). Viruses cause the majority of attacks of bronchitis and will precipitate most attacks of asthma. Some paediatricians have reverted recently to the older terms recurrent or wheezy bronchitis as most children with these features become free of symptoms by the age of 5 years. Although the pathological processes and prognosis may differ between recurrent bronchitis and bronchial asthma, there is no clinical or laboratory method of distinguishing between them and treatment is the same.

After an episode of severe symptoms during an infection with respiratory syncytial virus (bronchiolitis), many children have recurrent episodes of cough and wheezing during the subsequent 4 years. It is not known whether the respiratory syncytial virus predisposes the child to recurrent respiratory symptoms or whether the child has a predisposition to produce severe symptoms with viral respiratory infections.

If there is a persistent cough lasting more than 3 weeks a chest radiograph should be performed to exclude persistent segmental or lobar collapse. A Mantoux test for tuberculosis and a sweat test to exclude cystic fibrosis should be performed, and plasma concentrations of immunoglobulins and IgG subclasses should be measured to exclude transient or permanent immune deficiencies.

Bronchopneumonia and segmental pneumonia

Pneumonia is acute inflammation of the lung alveoli. In bronchopneumonia the infection is spread throughout the bronchial tree whereas in segmental pneumonia it is confined to the alveoli in one segment or lobe. A raised respiratory rate at rest or indrawing of the intercostal spaces distinguishes pneumonia from bronchitis. The upper limit for a normal respiratory rate is related to age (Table 4.1). Cough, fever, and flaring of the alae nasi are usually present and there may be reduced breath sounds over the affected area as well as crackles. A chest radiograph, which is needed for every child with suspected pneumonia, may show extensive changes when there are no localizing signs in the chest (Figure 4.1). The radiograph may show an opacity confined to a single segment or lobe but there may be bilateral, patchy changes. Bacterial cultures of throat swabs and blood should be performed before treatment is started. Ideally, nasopharyngeal secretions should be studied virologically and virus antibody titres of serum collected in the acute and convalescent phases should be measured.

Children with pneumonia are best treated in hospital as they may need oxygen treatment. Antibiotics should be prescribed for all children with pneumonia, although a viral cause may be discovered later. If the child is not vomiting and not severely ill, oral erythromycin or amoxicillin is given. Instead of erythromycin another

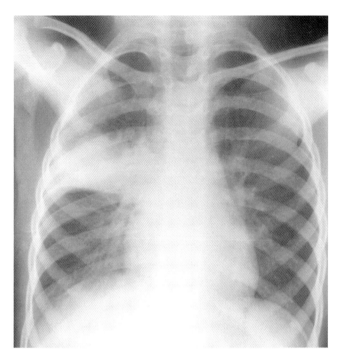

Figure 4.1 Segmental pneumonia.

macrolide, for example azithromycin or clarithromycin, may be given. Cefotaxime is given intravenously if the symptoms are severe, and erythromycin is added when failure to improve promptly suggests infection with *Mycoplasma* or *Chlamydia*. Antibiotic treatment can be modified when the results of bacterial cultures are available. Intravenous fluids may be needed.

A child who has had segmental or lobar pneumonia should be reviewed in the outpatient department after 1 month. If symptoms or abnormal signs are still present a chest radiograph should be performed to exclude a foreign body.

Whooping cough

Young infants receive no protective immunity to whooping cough from their mothers and have the highest incidence of complications. Immunization is directed at increasing herd immunity and reducing the exposure of infants to older children who have the disease.

Diagnosis

Whooping cough is difficult to diagnose during the first 7–14 days of the illness (catarrhal phase), when there is a short dry cough at night (Figure 4.2). Later, bouts of 10–20 short dry coughs occur day and night; each is on the same high note or rises in pitch. A long attack of coughing is followed by a sharp indrawing of breath, which may produce the crowing sound or whoop. Some children, especially babies, with *Bordetella pertussis* infection never develop the whoop. Feeding with crumbly food often provokes a coughing spasm, which may culminate in vomiting. Afterwards there is a short period when the child can be fed again without provoking coughing. In uncomplicated cases there are no abnormal respiratory signs.

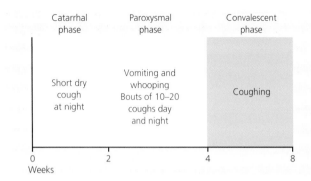

Figure 4.2 Phases of whooping cough.

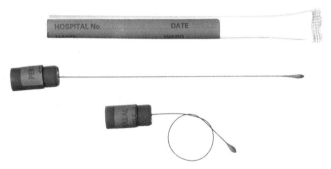

Figure 4.3 Per nasal swab for culture of *Bordetella pertussis*.

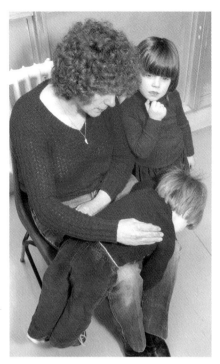

Figure 4.4 Chest physiotherapy.

The most important differential diagnosis in infants is bronchiolitis, which is usually caused by the respiratory syncytial virus and which produces epidemics of winter cough in infants less than 1 year. For the first few days there may be only bouts of vibratory rasping cough. Later, wheezes or crackles may be heard in the chest or there may be no abnormal signs. The infant either deteriorates or improves rapidly within a few days. Older siblings or the parents infected with the virus may have a milder illness. Other viruses may cause acute bronchitis with coughing but there are seldom more than two coughs at a time.

A properly taken per nasal swab plated promptly on a specific medium should reveal *B. pertussis* in most patients with whooping cough during the first few weeks of the illness (Figure 4.3). A blood lymphocyte count of 10×10^9/L or more with normal erythrocyte sedimentation rate suggests whooping cough. The diagnosis may be confirmed in infants with a clinical diagnosis late in the illness by blood antibody tests to *B. pertussis*.

Management

If the diagnosis is suspected in the catarrhal phase (usually because a sibling has had recognizable whooping cough) a 10-day course of erythromycin, or another macrolide, may be given to the child and to other children in the home. Parents must be warned that an antibiotic may shorten the course of the disease only in the early stages and is unlikely to affect established illness. Vomiting can be treated by giving soft, not crumbly, food or small amounts of fluid hourly.

No medicine reliably reduces the cough. Oral salbutamol has been used, but may disturb sleep. In severe cases, mothers can be taught to give physiotherapy, which may help to clear secretions, especially before the infant goes to sleep (Figure 4.4). An attack may be stopped by a gentle slap on the back.

The threshold for admission to hospital should be lower for children aged less than 6 months. Convulsions and cyanosis during coughing attacks are absolute indications for admission to an isolation cubicle. Parents often become exhausted by sleep loss and arranging for different members of the family to sleep with the child will give the mother a respite. The cough usually lasts for 8–12 weeks and may recur when the child has any new viral respiratory infection during the subsequent year. If the child is generally ill or the cough has not improved after 6 weeks, a chest radiograph should be performed to exclude bronchopneumonia or lobar collapse, which need treatment with physiotherapy and antibiotics. Long-term effects on the lung, such as bronchiectasis, are rare in developed countries.

The infant will not be infective for other children after about 4 weeks from the beginning of the illness or about 2 days after erythromycin is started. The incubation period is about 7 days and contacts who have no symptoms 2 weeks after exposure have usually escaped infection.

Tuberculosis

Tuberculosis (TB) is a major problem in developing countries and is increasing in prevalence in inner city areas. Children usually contract the infection by inhaling airborne droplets containing *Mycobacterium tuberculosis* from an adult. Most children with TB are identified because they are contacts of an affected adult. The bacteria enter the lungs, tonsils or small intestine and cause enlargement of the adjacent lymph nodes or spread to the blood. The infection may be carried to the meninges, bones, joints, kidneys, and pericardium. The main symptoms are prolonged fever (more than

10 days), chronic cough, malaise, and weight loss. The signs in the lungs may include pneumonia or a pleural effusion.

The diagnosis is confirmed by a chest radiograph and an intradermal injection of tuberculin purified protein derivative (PPD), which is called the Mantoux test. The injection site is checked for swelling 2 days later. Gastric washings may be cultured. Treatment consists of a combination of drugs for 6 months. It is essential that all the doses are given to avoid the emergence of strains of *M. tuberculosis* that are resistant to standard treatment.

Immunization against TB is given in the neonatal period with an attenuated vaccine (BCG) to infants at high risk. These families are from areas of high prevalence of TB. High risk includes a close relative or contact of the family who has received, or is receiving, treatment for TB in the previous 10 years. Also, those with parents or grandparents born in countries with a high prevalence of TB receive the vaccine. The vaccine produces a papule that enlarges over a few weeks and may ulcerate. It heals after about 8 weeks leaving a scar.

Recurrent respiratory infections

Although all doctors concerned with children are familiar with the catarrhal child, the exact pathology of the condition is unknown and it is called by many names – postnasal discharge, perennial rhinitis, or recurrent bronchitis. These children have an increased incidence of colds, tonsillitis, and acute otitis media. Recurrent episodes of symptoms such as fever, nasal discharge, and cough are most common during the second half of the first year of life, the first 2 years at nursery school, and the first 2 years at primary school. Recurrent viral or bacterial infections contracted from siblings or fellow pupils may be important, but the considerable differences between the behaviour of children in the same family suggest the possibility of a temporary immunological defect. During the winter several of these individual episodes may appear to join together to form an illness that lasts several months. On direct questioning, the mother will have observed a definite remission, if only for a few days between distinct episodes. If there are no remissions, especially if there has been vomiting, whooping cough should be considered.

Various treatments including nasal drops and oral preparations of antihistamines are given with little effect. A chest radiograph should be performed to exclude persistent segmental or lobar collapse. A sweat test should be carried out to exclude cystic fibrosis and plasma immunoglobulin studies should be conducted to exclude

rare syndromes. A Mantoux test should be considered, although interpretation may be difficult if the infant has received the BCG (see opposite).

Recurrent bronchitis

Two separate episodes of acute bronchitis may occur in a normal child in a year. If attacks are more frequent at any age, bronchial asthma should be considered. Viruses cause most attacks of bronchitis and will precipitate most attacks of bronchial asthma. Some paediatricians have reverted recently to the older terms recurrent or wheezy bronchitis, as most children with these features become free of symptoms by the age of 5. Although the pathological processes and prognosis may differ between recurrent bronchitis and bronchial asthma, there is no clinical or laboratory method of distinguishing between them and treatment is the same.

After an episode of severe symptoms during an infection with respiratory syncytial virus (bronchiolitis), many children have recurrent episodes of cough and wheezing during the subsequent 4 years. It is not known whether the respiratory syncytial virus predisposes the child to recurrent respiratory symptoms or whether the child has a predisposition to produce severe symptoms with viral respiratory infections. If there is a persistent or recurrent cough, a chest radiograph should be performed to exclude persistent segmental or lobar collapse. A Mantoux test for TB and a sweat test to exclude cystic fibrosis should be performed and plasma concentrations of immunoglobulins and IgG subclasses should be measured to exclude transient or permanent immune deficiencies.

The management of recurrent bronchitis or bronchial asthma is the same (see p. 24). For infants with mild symptoms a bronchodilatator can be given by a small spacer device with a face mask or by air pump and nebulizer. Infants with severe or frequent episodes can be given an inhaled steroid as a prophylactic drug for 6 weeks and the course can be extended to 6 months if there is an improvement in symptoms. Prophylactic drugs can be given with a small spacer device or by an air pump and nebulizer. If infants are receiving both a bronchodilatator and a prophylactic drug, the dose of bronchodilatator should be given just before the prophylactic drug.

Further reading

Prescribing of antibiotics for self-limiting respiratory tract infections in adults and children in primary care. NICE Clinical Guidelines, July 2008: CG 69. (www.NICE.org.uk)

CHAPTER 5

Tonsillitis and Otitis Media

Bernard Valman

Northwick Park Hospital and Imperial College London, UK

OVERVIEW

- Upper respiratory tract infections become more common after the age of 1 year, especially when starting to attend nursery or school. As preschool children have about six upper respiratory infections a year, these problems are extremely common.

- In the child the pharynx, tonsils, and middle ear are close together and it may seem arbitrary to divide them anatomically and prescribe separate treatment for each area (Figure 5.1). Although failing to give specific treatment for acute tonsillitis rarely results in sequelae, lack of treatment of acute otitis media may lead to bursting of the drum and a chronic discharge.

Tonsillitis and pharyngitis

In children aged less than 3 years the most common presenting features of tonsillitis are fever and refusal to eat, but a febrile convulsion may occur at the onset. Older children may complain of a sore throat or enlarged cervical lymph nodes, which may or may not be painful. Viral and bacterial causes cannot be distinguished clinically as a purulent follicular exudate may be present in both. Ideally, a throat swab should be sent to the laboratory before starting treatment to determine a bacterial cause for the symptoms and to help to indicate the pathogens currently in the community. If there has been a recurrence of group A haemolytic streptococci in outbreaks of sore throat, a more liberal use of penicillin is justified during this period. As this organism is the only important bacterium causing tonsillitis, penicillin is the drug of choice and the only justification for using another antibiotic is a convincing history of hypersensitivity to penicillin. In that case the alternative is erythromycin or another macrolide. In the absence of an outbreak of group A streptococcus infection the indication for oral penicillin is fever or severe systemic symptoms. The drug should be continued for at least 10 days if a streptococcal infection is confirmed. Parents often stop the drug after a few days as the symptoms have often abated and the medicine is unpalatable. The organism is not eradicated unless a full 10-day course is given.

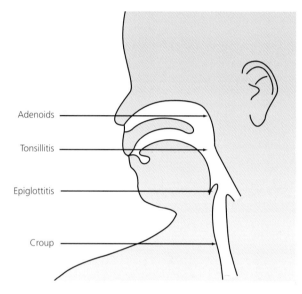

Figure 5.1 Sites of infection in respiratory tract.

Viral infections often produce two peaks on the temperature chart. An extensive, thick, white, shaggy exudate on the tonsils (sometimes invading the pharynx) suggests infectious mononucleosis, and a full blood count, examination of the blood film, and a Monospot test are indicated. A membranous exudate on the tonsils suggests diphtheria and an urgent expert opinion should be sought.

Fluids, ice cream, yogurt, or jelly can be given while there is dysphagia, and regular paracetamol or ibuprofen during the first 24–48 hours reduces fever and discomfort.

A peritonsillar abscess (quinsy) is now extremely rare. It displaces the tonsil medially so that the swollen soft palate obscures the tonsil and the uvula is displaced across the midline. The advice of an otolaryngology surgeon is needed urgently.

Acute otitis media

Pain is the main symptom of acute otitis media and is one of the reasons why a child wakes crying in the night. If the otitis media is bilateral the child has difficulty in locating the site of the pain. The pain is relieved if the drum ruptures. Viruses cause over half of cases of acute otitis media, but a viral or bacterial origin cannot

ABC of One to Seven, 5th edition. Edited by B. Valman. © 2010 Blackwell Publishing, ISBN: 978-1-4051-8105-1.

be distinguished clinically. The most common bacteria are pneumococci, group A haemolytic streptococci, and *Haemophilus influenzae*.

Children are often fascinated by the light of the auriscope, and the auriscope speculum can be placed on a doll's ear or the child's forearm for reassurance. Gentleness is essential and the speculum should never be pushed too far into the external meatus because this causes discomfort. If the pinna is pulled gently outwards to open the meatal canal the tympanic membrane is visible with the tip of a speculum only as far as the outer end of the meatus. In early cases of otitis media there are dilated vessels on the upper and posterior part of the drum (Figure 5.2). Later the tympanic membrane becomes congested and bulging and the light reflex becomes less clear. In severe cases of otitis media there may be bullous formation on the drum. This may cause acute pain initially, is not associated with a particular organism, and calls for no treatment apart from that of the acute otitis media. Swelling or tenderness behind the pinna should always be sought as mastoiditis may be easily missed.

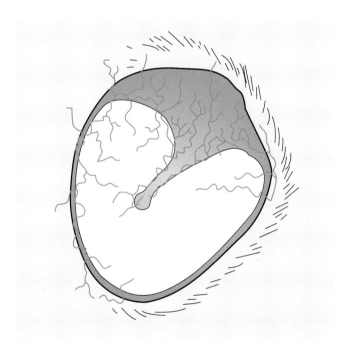

Figure 5.2 Appearance of drum in acute otitis media.

Recent research suggests that if there is no fever or systemic illness antibiotics should not be given initially. If there is no improvement after 48 hours a course of amoxicillin is given. If there is no improvement in the symptoms or appearance of the drum after a further 2–3 days another antibiotic should be substituted. Amoxicillin with clavulanic acid or cephalexin are second line drugs. There is no evidence that any form of ear drops is helpful in acute otitis media with an intact drum. Antibiotics should be given for 5 days and the ears examined again before the course is stopped. Three-day courses of antibiotics in a high dose may be as effective as longer courses.

Ideally, a hearing test should be performed 3 months after each attack of acute otitis media to detect residual deafness and secretory otitis media (glue ear). One study showed that, after the first attack of acute otitis media in infants that was treated with antimicrobial agents, 40% had no middle ear effusion after 1 month and 90% after 3 months.

The most appropriate hearing test varies with age (Table 5.1). The most accurate type of hearing test uses pure tones presented to children through earphones. Children signal that they have heard the sound by a prearranged sign such as putting a block into a cup. Children less than about 3 years old are not able to cooperate for this test and simple distraction tests are used, but considerable skill is needed and interpretation may be difficult. Adequate hearing for speech development is present if the hearing impairment is less than 20 decibels (Figure 5.3).

If three attacks of acute otitis media occur within 3 months and the drum has a normal appearance between attacks, a prophylactic drug should be considered. The most suitable drug is amoxicillin given at half the standard 24-hour dose in the evening only. This treatment is given for 3 months, and several studies have shown that the incidence of further attacks is reduced during that period. If the appearance of the drums does not return to normal after a 5-day course of treatment for acute otitis media the possibility of secretory otitis media should be considered.

Secretory otitis media

Secretory otitis media may be discovered during a routine hearing test. It may be found as a result of impaired hearing shown after an attack of acute otitis media. The insidious onset of this problem may result in the child presenting at school with a behaviour

Table 5.1 Appropriate hearing tests for age.

Test	Age	Procedure
Otoacoustic emissions	Any age	Sounds transmitted from generator to inner ear by device in ear. Echo is recorded
Auditory brainstem response	Any age	Device in ear makes sounds and the response of the 8th nerve is recorded from scalp electrodes
Distraction	6–18 months	Infant turns head to various noise stimuli
Visual reinforcement audiometry	6–32 months	Sounds presented through earphones or speakers and child is trained to turn to sound with a reward
Tympanometry (part of evaluation but not strictly a hearing test)	Any age	Tests mobility of drum and detects middle ear disease

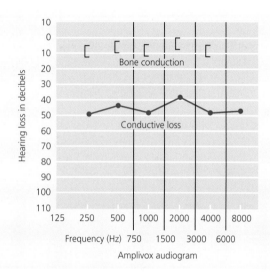

Amplivox audiogram

Figure 5.3 Audiogram in middle ear effusion.

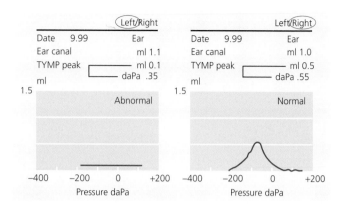

Figure 5.4 Tympanogram.

problem, slow learning, or periods of 'switching off' during lessons, which may be misinterpreted as petit mal. Hearing may fluctuate; some weeks it may be normal but at other times severely impaired. Routine screening tests may be performed during the good period and produce a false sense of security.

Fluid, often of glue-like consistency, fills the middle ear cavity in glue ear. This fluid reduces the movements of the tympanic membrane, resulting in hearing impairment. The cause is unknown, but it has been suggested that the middle ear fluid is unable to drain along the eustachian tube into the nasopharynx because of obstruction of the tube by mucopus or oedema.

The tympanic membrane can show a variety of abnormalities. There may be dilated vessels along the handle of the malleus and round the periphery of the drum, and they may radiate over the surface. The membrane may be normal in colour, pale amber, slate, or dark blue depending on the nature of the middle ear fluid.

If secretory otitis media is suspected the child should be seen by an otolaryngology surgeon. After the clinical examination a hearing test and tympanometry are performed (Figure 5.4). This test measures the movements of the drum by a special probe in the external auditory meatus. If the results of the tympanometry are abnormal it must be repeated after 6 weeks or 3 months, as a single observation is unreliable. The surgeon usually waits 3 months in the hope that the effusion will diminish or resolve. Previously, oral antihistamines and decongestant nose drops were given to improve eustachian tube drainage. Studies have shown that oral antihistamines have no clinical value and there is no evidence that nose drops are effective. If appreciable hearing loss (more than 20 decibels) and the effusion persist, myringotomy is performed under general anaesthesia (Box 5.1). The effusion is aspirated and a grommet may be inserted through the incision (Figures 5.5 and 5.6). This allows air into the middle ear, a role eventually resumed by the eustachian tube. The insertion of grommets is avoided unless there is good evidence of delay in speech development or that the duration of the effusion has been long. Grommets may cause scarring of the drum and the long-term effects of this complication are not known.

Box 5.1 **Advice for parents before grommet insertion**

What are grommets?
Grommets are small plastic tubes that allow air to enter the middle ear. First, we make a small cut in the ear drum and take out any fluid in the middle ear. The grommet is then inserted into the ear drum.

Going to hospital
You will be asked to bring your child to hospital a few days before the operation, for a day. This is so that the doctor can see if your child is fit for the operation, whether he or she still needs it and to perform any tests, such as blood or hearing tests, that might be needed. The anaesthetist may also see your child that day.

Going home from hospital
We will give you an advice sheet and explain it to you before you leave. Please ask any questions you may have.
We will make an outpatient appointment for you, usually after 6 weeks, to recheck your child's hearing. After that we will check every 6 months that the grommets are still working.

Will the grommets need to be removed?
Grommets usually fall out as the eardrum heals. This takes anywhere between 6 months and 2 years. They will work their way out of the ear canal with the wax. Usually you will not notice that they have come out. Sometimes, though, they will need another operation to remove them.

Will they need to be replaced?
Most children's ear problems are put right with one set of grommets. However, some children will need to have more put in.

General advice
You do need to protect your child's ears with ear plugs or cotton wool when bathing or washing the hair. Children with grommets can start to swim again after 6 weeks but must not dive or swim underwater.
Children with grommets are quite safe to travel by air. There is no risk of the grommet being knocked out in play or contact sports.

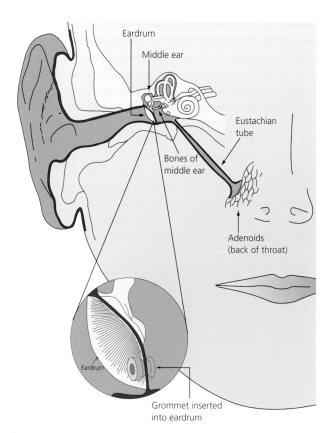

Figure 5.5 Grommet inserted in eardrum.

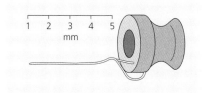

Figure 5.6 Grommet.

The grommet usually becomes blocked about 6–9 months after insertion. It is gradually extruded and falls out between 2 months and 2 years after insertion. The incision heals spontaneously. Glue ear sometimes recurs and the grommet may need to be inserted several times. Swimming may start 6 weeks after the insertion of grommets but diving or swimming underwater should be avoided. The value of adenoidectomy has been confirmed by controlled trials, and this procedure is often performed when grommets are inserted.

By the age of 7 or 8 years children who have had secretory otitis media usually have healthy ears and hearing in the normal range. This occurs as part of the natural history of the problem and is not related to the treatment. This means that, provided that the child with secretory otitis media has adequate hearing for his education, no medical or surgical treatment is needed. Apart from pure tone audiometry discussed above, the best test of adequate hearing is the level of speech development, and if appreciable hearing loss is detected or suspected, speech should be assessed and monitored regularly by a speech therapist. Children with secretory otitis media may have another factor, such as intellectual impairment or social deprivation, as the main cause of delay in their speech development.

Indications for tonsillectomy

If bacterial infection of the tonsils is suspected because there is pus on the tonsils and if group A haemolytic streptococci are grown from swabs more than three times a year in 2 consecutive years, tonsillectomy may be indicated. Many paediatricians would consider that these criteria are not stringent enough, although tonsillectomy would be a rare operation even if these less stringent criteria were followed. An absolute indication for tonsillectomy is such gross enlargement of the tonsils that they meet in the midline between attacks of infection and cause stridor or apnoea during sleep. During episodes of apnoea the blood oxygen saturation falls, and this can be detected by monitoring with a cutaneous oxymeter during overnight observation. Another indication is recurrent febrile convulsions associated with attacks of definite follicular tonsillitis.

Indications for adenoidectomy

Children with secretory otitis media (glue ear) should be seen by an otolaryngology surgeon. As well as aspiration of the middle ear and the insertion of a grommet, adenoidectomy is usually considered. If the surgeon considers that adenoidal tissue encroaches on the nasopharyngeal orifice of the eustachian tube he may perform an adenoidectomy. Partial nasal obstruction causing snoring at night and mouth breathing during the day with recurrent sore throat may be an indication for adenoidectomy, although there is a high rate of spontaneous cure if the parents can be persuaded to wait.

Further reading

Block CL. Searching for the Holy Grail of acute otitis media. *Arch Dis Child* 2006; **91**: 959–961.

Ludman H, Bradley P. *ABC of ENT*, 5th edn. BMJ, London, 2007.

CHAPTER 6

Stridor

Bernard Valman

Northwick Park Hospital and Imperial College London, UK

OVERVIEW

- Stridor is noisy breathing caused by obstruction in the pharynx, larynx, or trachea. It may be distinguished from partial obstruction of the bronchi by the absence of wheezes.

- Although most cases are caused by acute laryngitis and may resolve with the minimum of care, similar features may be caused by a foreign body or acute epiglottitis and may cause sudden death.

- Stridor is recognized as one of the most ominous signs in childhood. Any doctor should be able to recognize the sound over the telephone and arrange to see the child immediately (see Chapter 25).

- Examination of the throat may precipitate total obstruction of the airway and should be attempted only in the presence of an anaesthetist and facilities for intubation.

History and management

A glance at the child will show whether urgent treatment is needed or whether there is time for a detailed history to be taken. The doctor needs to know when the symptoms started and whether there is nasal discharge or cough. Choking over food, especially peanuts, or the abrupt onset of symptoms after playing alone with small objects suggests that a foreign body is present.

During the taking of the history and the examination the parent or carer should remain close and be encouraged to hold and to talk to the child. All unpleasant procedures such as venepuncture should be avoided. This reduces the possibility of struggling, which may precipitate complete airway obstruction. Agitation and struggling raise the peak flow rate and move secretions, which results in increased hypoxia and the production of more secretions.

Acute laryngotracheitis

Acute laryngitis causes partial obstruction of the larynx. It is characterized by inspiratory and expiratory stridor, cough, and hoarseness. The laryngeal obstruction is caused by oedema, spasm, and secretions. Affected children are usually aged 6 months to 3 years, and the symptoms are most severe in the early hours of the morning. Recession of the intercostal spaces indicates appreciable obstruction and cyanosis or drowsiness shows that total obstruction of the airway is imminent.

Complete airway obstruction may occur during examination of the throat of a child with stridor. The examination should be attempted only in the presence of an anaesthetist and facilities for intubation, preferably in the anaesthetic room of the operating theatre.

A child often improves considerably after inhaling steam, which is provided easily by turning on the hot taps in the bathroom at home. A single dose of dexamethasone or prednisolone is given. Mild cases may be treated successfully at home using this method but the child must be visited every few hours to determine whether the condition is deteriorating and the child needs to be admitted to hospital. Continuous stridor, cyanosis, drowsiness, or recession demand urgent hospital admission. Before transfer, dexamethasone or prednisolone is given. In hospital dexamethasone is given orally or by injection, or budesonide is given by nebulizer and is repeated after 12 hours (Figure 6.1). There is usually an improvement within an hour. Oxygen with humidity can be given. If the symptoms are severe or the child deteriorates despite the steroids, nebulized adrenaline is given and repeated after 30 minutes if necessary.

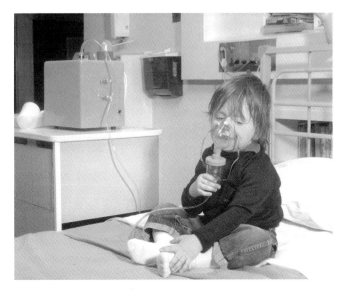

Figure 6.1 Pump and nebulizer.

ABC of One to Seven, 5th edition. Edited by B. Valman. © 2010 Blackwell Publishing, ISBN: 978-1-4051-8105-1.

Monitoring in a high dependency or intensive care unit is needed to detect a possible recurrence of an obstruction. Hypoxaemia or thirst may cause restlessness and should be corrected and sedatives avoided. Obstruction only rarely needs to be relieved by passing an endotracheal tube. A cutaneous oximeter can provide an early warning of hypoxia.

Acute laryngotracheitis is usually caused by a viral infection and therefore infants with mild symptoms do not need antibiotics. In a few cases *Staphylococcus aureus* or *Haemophilus influenzae* is present and the associated septicaemia makes the child appear very ill. Bacterial infection is characterized by plaques of debris and pus on the surface of the trachea, partially obstructing it, just below the vocal cords. If bacterial infection is suspected cefotaxime is given intravenously. Acute epiglottitis (see below) and acute laryngitis may be indistinguishable clinically as stridor and progressive upper airway obstruction are the main features of both.

Acute epiglottitis

Children with epiglottitis are usually aged over 2 years; drooling and dysphagia are common, and the child usually wants to sit upright. When the obstruction is very severe the stridor becomes ominously quieter. There is usually an associated septicaemia with *H. influenzae*.

If epiglottitis is suspected the child should be transferred urgently to hospital. Facilities for intubation must be available when the throat is examined because the examination may cause complete airway obstruction. The epiglottis is red and swollen. Acute epiglottitis has a high mortality. Some units have found a lateral radiograph of the neck helpful in distinguishing between acute laryngitis and acute epiglottitis (Figure 6.2). The films must be taken in the intensive care unit with the child in the upright position in the presence of a doctor skilled in intubation. As it is impossible to distinguish clinically between infection with *H. influenzae* and a viral infection, cefotaxime should be given intravenously.

Other causes and emergency management of foreign bodies

Even if the symptoms have settled and there are no abnormal signs, a history of the onset of sudden choking or coughing can never be ignored. A radiograph of the neck and chest should be taken and

may show a hypertranslucent lung on the side of a foreign body, a shift of the mediastinum, or, less commonly, collapse of part of the lung or a radiopaque foreign body. The radiograph may be considered normal. Bronchoscopy may be needed to exclude a foreign body even if the chest radiograph appears to be normal. Stridor in a child who has had scalds or burns or has inhaled steam from a kettle suggests that intubation or tracheostomy may be needed urgently.

If the cause of stridor is likely to be a foreign body below the larynx the object should be removed immediately by a thoracic surgeon in the main or emergency operating theatre.

If the object is above the larynx and if an otolaryngology surgeon or anaesthetist is not immediately available no attempt should be made to look at the mouth or throat or remove the object, as the struggling that may follow can impact the object and prove fatal. The child should remain in the position he finds most comfortable, which is usually upright. Forceful attempts to make the child lie flat, for example for a radiograph, may result in complete airway obstruction.

If there is a definite history of aspiration of a foreign body and symptoms are increasing, or lifting the chin has failed to open the airway of an apnoeic patient, an attempt should be made to expel the foreign body. Back blows or chest thrusts are given in an infant (Figures 6.3 and 6.4) and the Heimlich manoeuvre

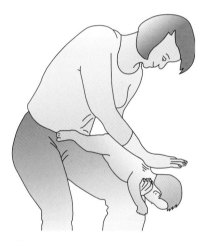

Figure 6.3 Back blows.

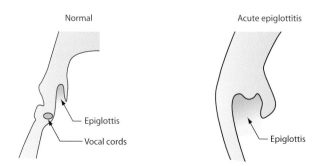

Figure 6.2 Radiological appearance of normal epiglottis and acute epiglottitis.

Radiographic appearances

Normal

Acute epiglottitis

Epiglottis

Vocal cords

Epiglottis

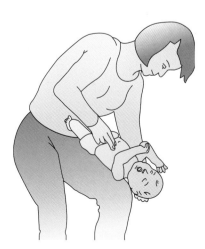

Figure 6.4 Chest thrusts.

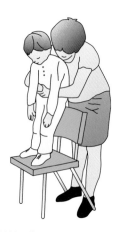

Figure 6.5 Heimlich manoeuvre.

involving manual compression of the upper abdomen, raising intra-abdominal pressure, in the older child (Figure 6.5).

Further reading

Mackway-Jones K, Molyneux E, Phillips B, Wieteska S, eds. *Advanced Paediatric Life Support*, 4th edn. Blackwell Publishing, Oxford, 2004.

CHAPTER 7

Asthma

Bernard Valman

Northwick Park Hospital and Imperial College London, UK

OVERVIEW

- Asthma should be suspected in any child who wheezes, ideally heard by a health professional on auscultation. The diagnosis is made clinically with confirmation by peak flow measurements where there is uncertainty in the older child.

- The symptoms of asthma are caused by narrowing of the bronchi and bronchioles by mucosal swelling and contraction of the muscle in their walls, with viscid secretion obstructing the lumen (Figure 7.1). The muscle contraction is reversible by a bronchodilatator such as salbutamol which is a β_2-agonist. Corticosteroids reduce mucosal oedema and secretions.

- In most children with asthma there are no symptoms or abnormal signs between acute attacks, and lung function tests, unless performed before and after exercise, are normal.

- Asthma is the most common chronic disease of childhood and it affects about 10% of schoolchildren. About 80% of children with asthma have the first symptoms before the age of 5 years and at least half will stop having attacks when they become adults.

- Prophylactic drugs and better methods of administering them have resulted in many children with asthma being completely free of symptoms.

- Treatment needs to be reviewed regularly to ensure that the child is receiving the minimum doses of drugs that produces optimal control.

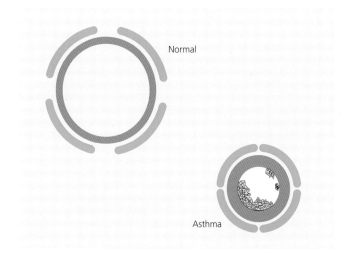

Figure 7.1 Structural changes in asthma.

Diagnosis

Asthma should be suspected if there is recurrent cough, wheezing, and shortness of breath, especially after exercise or during the night. Improvement with a bronchodilator is helpful evidence but is not specific for asthma. The first attack may occur at any age, but to avoid many children with an acute lower respiratory tract infection being labelled as having asthma it is preferable to wait until three episodes have occurred within a year before confirming the diagnosis. There is no clinical or laboratory method of distinguishing between acute bronchial infection and asthma. Wheezes may be heard in the chest during and between attacks of asthma, but there may be no abnormal signs despite repeated examinations. The absence of night cough is the best evidence that treatment is adequate. The length of absences from school, as well as the number of hospital admissions, give an indication of the severity of the problem. Details of previous drug treatments may help to avoid the repetition of failures.

Features not commonly found in asthma may indicate an alternative diagnosis. Cough present from birth, a family history of unusual chest disease, persistent wet cough, diarrhoea, or failure to thrive suggest cystic fibrosis (see p. 41). Excessive vomiting suggests the possibility of gastro-oesophageal reflux with or without aspiration. Sudden onset suggests inhalation of a foreign body.

Most children with recurrent cough but no wheeze do not have asthma. As wheeze may not be recognized, a 2-week course of asthma treatment may be given but should be stopped if there is no improvement and the dose should not be increased. The cough is induced by a viral infection or an irritant, such as smoke, affecting airways with increased cough receptor sensitivity. The increased sensitivity is temporary and no medication reduces it.

ABC of One to Seven, 5th edition. Edited by B. Valman. © 2010 Blackwell Publishing, ISBN: 978-1-4051-8105-1.

Assessment

A detailed history should be taken of exposure to household pets or other animals which may belong to friends or relatives. Severe symptoms or hayfever at a particular time of the year may incriminate pollen. Skin tests are no longer performed for most patients with asthma as they rarely lead to a change in treatment. Skin tests tend to be negative under the age of 5 years and also when the child is taking steroids. Exposure to tobacco smoke is associated with an increase in symptoms and should be avoided.

The single most useful test is the peak flow reading, which can be measured in children older than 5 years using the low range (30–400 L/min) mini-Wright peak flow meter (Figure 7.2). Normal ranges are related to the height of the child but the child's own best performance during remission is the best guide for future management (Figure 7.3). In asthma peak flow varies greatly throughout the day, being lowest in the early morning and shortly after exercise. This exercise can be of any type. A fall in peak expiratory flow rate of 15% or more after exercise or a similar rise with a bronchodilatator confirms the diagnosis. About 10% of children with asthma have a normal response to these tests. Regular peak flow reading and completion of a standard diary card of symptoms may be helpful in assessing the severity of the problem and the response to treatment (Figure 7.4).

A chest radiograph is taken at the initial assessment to help exclude alternative diagnoses such as cystic fibrosis, immune deficiencies and other causes of bronchiectasis, infection including tuberculosis, congenital lung malformations, and inhaled foreign body. If a child has once had a normal radiograph further films are usually not helpful.

The importance of psychological factors in inducing attacks of asthma is difficult to assess, although stresses caused by absence from school, disruption of the family, and conflicting advice are inevitable in the severely affected child. The problem of the child who has had a recent increase in attacks or who is poorly controlled despite apparently adequate treatment should be discussed by the paediatrician with a child psychiatrist. The help given by child psychiatrists may depend on their enthusiasm.

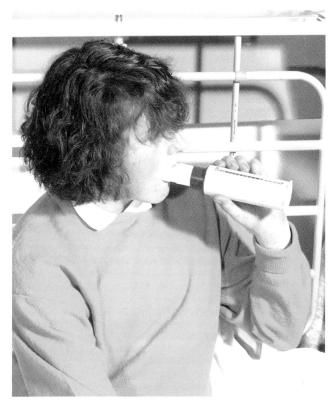

Figure 7.2 Wright peak flow meter.

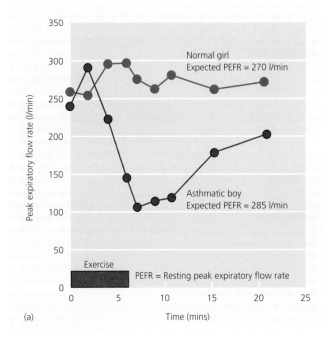

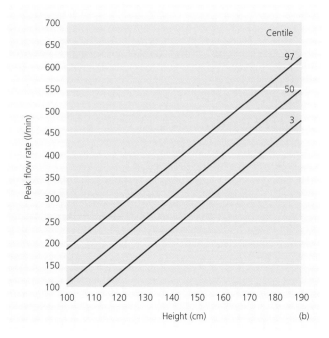

Figure 7.3 (a) Peak flow rates: related to exercise. (b) Peak flow rates: normal range.

		1	2	3	4	5	6	7	8	9	10

Date this card was started

1. WHEEZE LAST NIGHT

Good night ——————————— 0
Slept well but slightly wheezy ———— 1
Woke x 2-3 because of wheeze ———— 2
Bad night, awake most of time ———— 3

2. COUGH LAST NIGHT

None ——————————————— 0
Little ——————————————— 1
Moderately bad ————————— 2
Severe ——————————————— 3

3. WHEEZE TODAY

None ——————————————— 0
Little ——————————————— 1
Moderately bad ————————— 2
Severe ——————————————— 3

4. ACTIVITY TODAY

Quite normal ————————— 0
Can only run short distance ———— 1
Limited to walking because of chest ———— 2
Too breatheless to walk ————— 3

5. NASAL SYMPTOMS

None ——————————————— 0
Mild ——————————————— 1
Moderate ————————————— 2
Severe ——————————————— 3

6. METER Best of 3 blows

Before breakfast medicines ————

Before bedtime medicines ————

7. DRUGS

Number of doses actually taken during the past 24 hours

Name of drug	Dose Prescribed

8. COMMENTS

Note if you see a doctor (D) or stay away from school (S) or work (W) because of your chest and anything else important such as an infection (I)

Figure 7.4 Diary chart of symptoms.

Allergen avoidance

A recent Cochrane review concluded that methods to reduce exposure to house dust mite allergens cannot be recommended in the treatment of asthma. This was based on 54 trials including 3000 patients and the authors considered the negative evidence so strong that further trials were unlikely to change the conclusion. The British Thoracic Society (BTS) asthma guideline does not recommend allergen avoidance but the US guidelines still do. Committed parents of a child with house dust allergy who wish to minimize exposure to house dust may be advised as follows. Complete avoidance of house dust is impossible, but feather pillows can be replaced by foam rubber pillows and the mattress can be completely enclosed in a plastic bag. It may be helpful for a damp duster to be used for wiping surfaces and for the affected child's rooms to be cleaned while he is in another part of the house. Vinyl floor covering can be used instead of carpets.

The importance of food in precipitating attacks and the value of exclusion diets in preventing symptoms are controversial. Some studies suggest that the following items have precipitated symptoms in specific children: orange and lemon squash, fried foods, nuts, and drinks containing ice or carbon dioxide. If parents have noted that symptoms are precipitated by a particular food it would seem reasonable to avoid that food for a limited trial period of 6 weeks, but the diet should be supervised by a paediatric dietitian.

Although food allergy may not be important in the aetiology of asthma, it is crucial to recognize that a child with a history of immediate food allergic reaction (anaphylaxis) is at much greater risk of death during subsequent exposure if he also has asthma. Foods particularly important to enquire about are peanuts and tree nuts, milk, eggs, fish, and shellfish.

Management

Aims

Effective treatment should allow the child to take part in all types of exercise and sport and there should be no symptoms either at night or during the day (Box 7.1). Absence from school should be minimal. There should be no early morning fall in expiratory peak flow rate. Relieving doses of bronchodilatators should be needed less than three times a week and growth should be normal. Changes in treatment are needed if these aims are not being achieved.

Action plan

The patients and their parents need to understand the condition, treatment, and how to respond to any changes (Box 7.2). They need to appreciate the use of inhaled drugs and peak flow meters and the difference between preventive and symptomatic treatment. A patient diary is helpful in assessing the effectiveness of treatment by monitoring symptoms, peak flow, and drug usage, and it can be supplemented by written guidelines on action to be taken by the parents if the symptoms change.

Drug treatment

Mild asthma causes symptoms that do not interfere with sleep or lifestyle or episodes of cough and wheeze less than once a month. Moderate asthma is either discrete attacks occurring no more often than once a week or more chronic symptoms that do not affect growth. Severe asthma can be defined as continuous cough or wheezing on most days or nights, or severe attacks requiring oral or intravenous steroids (Box 7.3).

Children with mild asthma should receive a β_2-agonist as needed rather than at regular intervals (BTS step 1). Inhaled steroids are added (BTS step 2) if any of the following are present:

- An acute attack during the previous 2 years;
- A β_2-agonist is used three times weekly or more;
- Waking at night occurs once or more each week.

The starting dose depends on the severity of asthma in that child but is usually 200 micrograms of beclometasone, or an equivalent drug, twice daily. The dose is reduced aiming for a once daily low dose which maintains control. The dose is reduced by 25–50% every 3–6 months if the child is free of symptoms.

Box 7.1 **Aims**

With effective treatment a child:
- Can play all sport and do all exercise
- Has no symptoms, day or night
- Has minimal absences from school
- Has no early morning fall in expiratory peak flow rate
- Needs bronchodilator relief less than three times a week
- Has normal growth

Box 7.2 **Action plan**

To ensure effective treatment children and parents should:
- Understand the condition
- Know the difference between preventive and symptomatic treatment
- Know how to use inhaled drugs and peak flow meters
- Monitor symptoms, peak flow, and drug usage in a patient diary
- Be given guidelines for action if the symptoms change

Box 7.3 **Drug treatment**

Mild asthma
- Symptoms do not interfere with sleep or lifestyle
- Episodes of cough or wheeze less than once a month
- Responds to bronchodilatator immediately

Moderate asthma
- Attacks less than once a week, or
- Chronic symptoms, do not affect growth or development

Severe asthma
- Continuous cough or wheeze most days or nights, or
- Severe attacks requiring oral or intravenous steroids

Children who are not well controlled with 200 micrograms of beclometasone and a short-acting β_2-agonist should have an assessment of compliance, inhaler technique, and possible trigger factors. The dose of beclometasone can be increased but should not exceed 400 micrograms per day as side effects (see below) are more likely at high doses. Children who are not well controlled on 400 micrograms per day of beclometasone should be referred to a paediatrician. If the paediatrician is satisfied with the diagnosis, compliance, and inhaler technique, a third drug will be added (BTS step 3). Those over the age of 5 years may be prescribed a long-acting β_2-agonist (LABA) and those under 5 years a leukotriene receptor antagonist (LTRA) in addition to an inhaled steroid. If this is inadequate all four drugs may be prescribed (BTS step 4: inhaled β-agonist, steroid, LABA, and oral LTRA).

Recent evidence shows that teenagers taking both inhaled LABA and steroids can use a combination inhaler as required rather than regularly twice daily. This is a major advance for this age group who have poor compliance with regular asthma dosing regimes. Any child taking prophylactic drugs should always have available a fast-acting bronchodilatator to treat acute attacks and to be used half an hour before vigorous exercise if the prophylactic drug is known to be ineffective. The recommendation in the UK from the Chief Medical Officer is that all patients requiring inhaled steroid prophylaxis are given annual influenza vaccination, but in practice this is usually only offered to children with severe asthma.

The selection of a route of administration that is appropriate to the age of the child is essential for effective treatment (Table 7.1). A common cause of failure to respond to an inhaled drug is lack of proper tuition, and it is helpful if a practice nurse or health visitor takes on this task for all the children in the practice. Bronchodilatator drugs can be given at any age, but they tend to be less effective in infants under the age of 18 months.

Metered dose inhalers should be prescribed for children only if the prescription is accompanied by repeated, thorough, and correct tuition (Figure 7.5). It is essential that the coordination of inspiration and release of the dose is checked. This delivery system should not be prescribed for children younger than 8 years unless it is accompanied by a spacer device with a valve system (Figure 7.6). This allows children of 2–3 years or older to use this form of treatment for all medications. Some younger infants may be able to use a spacer with a closely fitting face mask (Figure 7.7). During acute episodes children may not be able to move the valve and only a nebulizer will be appropriate.

For children and infants who are unable to cooperate with a spacer system, an electric pump and nebulizer are needed to provide an aerosol which is delivered with a face mask held near the

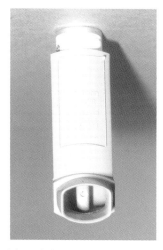

Figure 7.5 Metered dose inhaler.

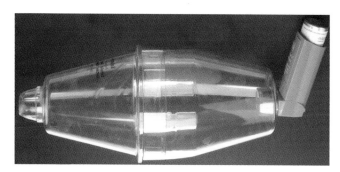

Figure 7.6 Metered dose inhaler with valved spacer.

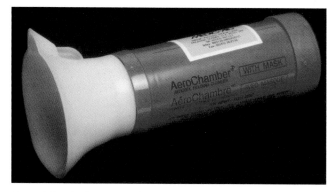

Figure 7.7 Valved spacer with face mask.

Table 7.1 Inhalation delivery systems.

Inhalation delivery system	Relieving treatment	Preventive treatment
Metered dose inhaler + valved spacer (with face mask for children younger than 5 years or with learning difficulties)	Salbutamol Terbutaline Ipratropium bromide	Beclometasone Budesonide Fluticasone Salmeterol Formoterol
Nebulizer and air compressor	Salbutamol Terbutaline Ipratropium bromide	Budesonide
Powder inhaler	Salbutamol (Accuhaler) Terbutaline (Turbohaler)	Budesonide (Turbohaler) Fluticasone (Accuhaler) Salmeterol (Accuhaler) Formoterol (Turbohaler)

Note: Combination inhalers are available of salmeterol and fluticasone (Seretide, manufactured by GlaxoSmithKline) or budesonide and formoterol (Symbicort, manufactured by AstraZeneca).

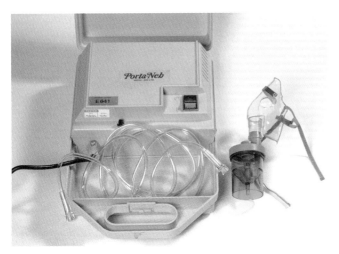

Figure 7.8 Pump with nebulizer.

Table 7.2 Clinical features for assessment of severity.

Acute severe	Life-threatening
Too breathless to talk or feed	Cyanosis
Pulse	
>120 beats/min aged >5 years	Poor respiratory effort
>130 beats/min aged 2–5 years	Confusion or coma
Respiratory rate	
>30 breaths/min aged >5 years	Silent chest
>50 breaths/min aged 2–5 years	Exhaustion

Box 7.4 Criteria for discharge from emergency department

- No symptoms
- Peak flow >75% of best value 1 hour after initial treatment
- Oximeter reading >94% in air
- Controlled on 3–4 hourly bronchodilator

---

child's face (Figure 7.8). The ideal volume of fluid for the nebulizer is 4 mL which should take 10 minutes to administer.

Where a β_2-agonist and inhaled steroid are used together, the β_2-agonist should be given first to increase the calibre of the airways. The use of regular, inhaled β_2-agonists more than three times a day has been implicated as a factor contributing to morbidity and deaths from asthma and it is advisable to minimize the use of regular β_2-agonists.

A few patients who are well controlled with prophylactic drugs need three to four courses of daily oral steroids each year during exacerbations. Each course should last 2–5 days and the dosage is 2 mg/kg/day prednisolone (maximum dose 40 mg/day). There is no need to taper off the doses. Oral steroids given are still needed for a few children who have failed to respond to all other forms of treatment, but these children should be under the close supervision of a paediatrician. Children who are receiving oral steroids or high doses of inhaled steroids may develop adrenal insufficiency which causes shock at the time of intercurrent acute infection. At present there is no reliable method of predicting this risk and normal growth does not exclude it. Other side effects include reduction in bone density, diabetes, and cataracts. Poor growth in height in a child with asthma may be a result of asthma that is inadequately controlled or a side effect of steroids in high doses.

Acute attacks of asthma

Viral infections are the most important precipitating cause of attacks of asthma, and antibiotics are therefore not indicated except for selected patients with severe attacks requiring hospital admission.

Each child with asthma should have a written plan for the emergency management of attacks. If an acute asthma attack does not respond quickly to the child's usual treatment at home, he will need urgent treatment with additional inhaled salbutamol or terbutaline aerosol. This can be given by a metered dose inhaler with a spacer or a face mask. If a nebulizer is used it should preferably have an oxygen supply. If the family doctor is not immediately available to provide this treatment the child should be seen in hospital. Delay in appreciating the severity of the attack or providing treatment can be fatal.

Drowsiness, cyanosis of the lips, and shortness of breath during speaking are signs of a severe attack (Table 7.2). The duration of the episode of asthma and details of the drugs taken previously should be noted, especially those taken during the preceding 24 hours.

Children with life-threatening asthma or oximeter readings <92% should receive high flow oxygen with a tightly fitting face mask or nasal cannula at sufficient flow to achieve normal saturations.

Up to 10 puffs (1000 micrograms of salbutamol) of a β_2-agonist is given every 30 minutes by a metered dose inhaler and spacer. A child in primary care should be transferred to hospital if there is no improvement after two doses and further doses should be given with oxygen on the journey. If the child does not accept the spacer, the bronchodilatator can be given with a nebulizer each hour.

Bronchodilatator drugs can be given to children of any age and are accepted if the mask is held by the mother and she talks to the child during treatment. The mother's presence calms the child. The condition has usually improved considerably before the dose is finished. Criteria for discharge are shown in Box 7.4.

Indications for admission are:

- Any feature of a life-threatening or fatal attack;
- Significant symptoms persisting after initial treatment;
- Pulse oximeter reading of <92% saturation after initial bronchodilatator treatment with air;
- <50% predicted peak flow rate or poor improvement after initial bronchodilatator treatment.

Treatment on admission

On the way to hospital the child should be encouraged to sit upright in the position that makes him most comfortable; this is usually with his elbows forward.

A further dose of nebulized β_2-agonist is given with continuous humidified oxygen. The adequacy of the concentration of oxygen in the blood is monitored by cutaneous oximetry. Failure to respond indicates the need for oral or intravenous steroids. The dose of oral

Box 7.5 **Treatment cascade**

- Inhaled β_2-agonist
- Inhaled β_2-agonist with oxygen
- Oral steroids and inhaled ipratropium bromide
- Intravenous salbutamol or aminophylline
- Intravenous magnesium sulphate
- Intubation and ventilation

prednisolone is 20 mg for children aged 2–5 years and 30–40 mg for those aged >5 years. If the child has been taking steroids before this episode the dose is 2 mg/kg body weight each day. The steroids are given for about 3 days and the dose is not tapered. The steroids take about 3 hours to be effective and the child may deteriorate during this period.

Inhaled ipratropium bromide is added to the next dose of inhaled salbutamol. If the attack is severe and the patient does not respond quickly to treatment, a chest radiograph should be performed to exclude pneumothorax or pneumonia.

If the child's condition is deteriorating, he should be admitted to the intensive care unit. Meanwhile, an intravenous salbutamol bolus (15 micrograms/kg over 20 minutes followed by an infusion of 1–5 micrograms/kg/min) and/or intravenous aminophylline are given. If the child has still not improved, a bolus of intravenous magnesium sulphate (40 mg/kg, maximum dose 2 g) is given over 20 minutes (Box 7.5).

Although bronchodilatator treatment may be effective within a few minutes, steroid treatment takes several hours to be effective. Deterioration may occur rapidly, and the same observer should see the patient at least every half hour. Arterial blood is taken for urgent estimations of oxygen and carbon dioxide concentrations, pH, plasma sodium, and potassium concentrations. Clinical deterioration despite maximum treatment is the main indication for intubation and ventilation.

Asthma in children under 2 years

The younger the infant the more difficult it is to diagnose and treat asthma. For those with mild to moderate asthma, salbutamol can be given with a metered dose inhaler, spacer, and face mask. As bronchodilatators are less effective in those under the age of 18 months, short courses of oral steroids should be considered at an early stage. Failure to respond quickly to a β_2-agonist is an indication to add inhaled ipratropium bromide to the inhaled β_2-agonist.

Discharge plans for all ages should include:

- Inhaler technique checked;
- Regular prophylactic treatment considered;
- Written emergency action plan given including:
  - use of bronchodilatator
  - methods of seeking urgent medical advice
  - indications for starting oral steroids
- Appointment with family doctor in 1 week and asthma clinic in 1 month.

Future prospects

Asthma treatment has improved considerably in recent years with new drugs (especially leukotriene antagonists and LABAs), and new treatment strategies (e.g. as required combination inhalers for teenagers). There has been less progress in understanding the aetiology and why asthma is becoming more common. Although prevention is still not foreseeable, there are new therapies becoming available such as monoclonal anti-IgE antibody for select patient groups.

Further reading

British Thoracic Society Scottish Intercollegiate Guidelines Network. British guideline on the management of asthma. *Thorax* 2008; **63** (Suppl IV): 1–121.

Gøtzsche PC, Johansen HK. House dust mite control measures for asthma. *Cochrane Database Syst Rev* 2008; Issue 2.

National Institute for Health and Clinical Excellence (NICE). *Inhaled Corticosteroids for the Treatment of Chronic Asthma in Children Under the Age of 12 Years.* NICE Technology Appraisal Guidance 131. NICE, London, 2007.

CHAPTER 8

Acute Abdominal Pain

Bernard Valman

Northwick Park Hospital and Imperial College London, UK

OVERVIEW

- At the beginning of an episode of abdominal pain it may be difficult to make an exact diagnosis. The picture will become clearer if the child is seen again after a few hours, but if this is not possible the child may have to be admitted to an ambulatory care unit (see Chapter 36) or hospital for observation.

- Many parents are worried that their child has acute appendicitis, and the responsibility for observing the child should not be left to the parents, who do not have the knowledge to make the right judgements.

- Although a definite diagnosis should be attempted it is essential to place the patient in one of the following groups:

  1 Surgical problem: admit;

  2 Chronic medical problem: arrange paediatric appointment;

  3 Gastroenteritis: manage at home or admit to an isolation cubicle of the ambulatory care (see Chapter 36) or paediatric unit depending on the severity of the illness;

  4 Acute non-specific abdominal pain;

  5 Cause uncertain: see again within a few hours or admit to hospital for observation.

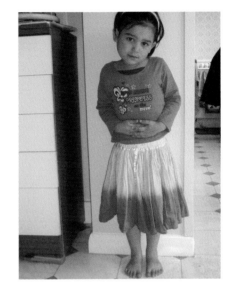

Figure 8.1 Taking history from child.

Surgical problems

Appendicitis may produce features suggestive of many other conditions and it may not be possible to make a firm diagnosis or to exclude it on one observation. If surgical intervention is a possibility the parents should be warned not to give their child any food or drink in the meantime as a general anaesthetic may be needed.

Although the parent gives the details of the history, it is important to obtain as much information as possible from the child directly (Figure 8.1). However, children under the age of 3 years may point to the abdomen as the site of pain when in fact the cause of the symptoms is in another area such as the throat. Abdominal tenderness can be observed even in small children, who may push away the examiner's hand.

The site and duration of the pain should be noted and whether previous attacks have occurred. The duration and severity of diarrhoea or vomiting should be noted. There may be fever, rash, or pain in the joints.

Appendicitis

The wall of the appendix is thinner in children than in adults; the omentum is less developed and perforation is often followed by generalized peritonitis. The child himself should be asked about his pain. Older children can often localize their pain accurately if they are asked to point to the pain with one finger (Figure 8.2). In acute appendicitis pain around the umbilicus often starts suddenly and is followed by vomiting. The pain may be intermittent or continuous and colicky or dull. It may be relieved during sleep. After a few hours, during which there may be some improvement, the pain moves to the right iliac fossa. In about one-quarter of patients the pain is in the right iliac fossa from the beginning. A child with appendicitis may have constipation or diarrhoea. Body temperature may be raised. The child usually lies still as the pain

ABC of One to Seven, 5th edition. Edited by B. Valman. © 2010 Blackwell Publishing, ISBN: 978-1-4051-8105-1.

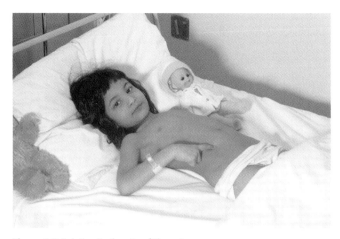

Figure 8.2 Pointing to the site of the pain.

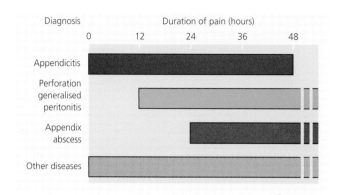

Figure 8.3 Complications of acute appendicitis related to the time of onset of pain.

is aggravated by movement. Movements of the abdominal wall during breathing are restricted.

Appendicitis is extremely difficult to diagnose in infants under 2 years old, and perforation often occurs before the diagnosis is made. Then the infant looks extremely ill and has considerable abdominal tenderness.

The bladder should be emptied before the abdomen is examined. The abdomen should be palpated gently with a warm hand or the bell end of a stethoscope, beginning in the *left* iliac fossa. Tenderness is detected by change of expression on the child's face, and is localized to the right iliac fossa before perforation. Guarding can be assessed only if the child is completely relaxed. Bowel sounds are reduced if perforation has already occurred. Rectal examination should be performed only once and it is better to leave it to the surgeon. Very gentle examination is necessary to determine local tenderness rectally. The fact that a rectal examination has not been performed should be recorded in the patient's notes.

If the appendix is situated in the pelvis or behind the caecum diagnosis is particularly difficult. Tenderness may be shown only on deep palpation and there may be diarrhoea or urinary symptoms, but there is no excess of pus cells in the urine microscopically.

A full physical examination should be performed to exclude disease in another organ, especially the respiratory system, as it may be responsible for the symptoms. The white cell count is not helpful and need not be considered as a routine test for children with suspected appendicitis. Microscopy of the urine should be carried out immediately if there is any doubt about the diagnosis, and chest radiography should be considered.

If a definite diagnosis cannot be made initially the child should be examined several times during the first 24 hours of pain, because perforation is more likely if the pain has been present for a longer period (Figure 8.3). These repeated examinations should be performed by the same doctor if possible. If the pain lasts longer than 48 hours the child is likely to have generalized peritonitis, an appendix abscess, or pain not related to the appendix. If an episode of pain lasts continuously for longer than 6 hours the patient should be examined again.

Acute appendicitis and the other diagnoses discussed below should be considered in every child with acute abdominal pain but

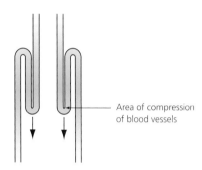

Figure 8.4 Compression of blood vessels in intussusception.

in most children the cause cannot be found. The final diagnosis has been termed 'acute non-specific abdominal pain' and suggestive features include intermittent central abdominal pain and tenderness without guarding lasting 24–36 hours. Sore throat, fever, or vomiting may be present. Clusters of cases suggest that there are infectious causes.

Intussusception

An intussusception is a partial or complete intestinal obstruction caused by invagination of a proximal portion of the gut into a more distal portion (Figure 8.4). It may occur at any age although the maximum incidence is at 3–11 months. An intussusception may be diagnosed easily in a child who has all the typical features, but these children are not common. The distinctive feature is the periodicity of the attacks, which may consist of severe screaming, drawing up of the legs, and severe pallor. Some episodes consist of pallor alone. The attack lasts a few minutes and then disappears, to recur about 20 minutes later, although attacks may be more frequent. One or two loose stools may be passed initially, suggesting a diagnosis of acute gastroenteritis. Bloodstained mucus may be passed rectally or shown by rectal examination but some patients pass no blood rectally. Between attacks the infant seems normal and there may be no abnormal signs apart from a palpable mass.

It is difficult to examine the abdomen during an attack because the child cries continuously, but between attacks a mass, most commonly in the right upper quadrant, can be felt in 70% of children with intussusception.

If surgical shock is present then rapid resuscitation should be carried out and intravenous fluids, including blood, given. Plain radiographs of the abdomen may show evidence of intestinal obstruction or a density in the area of the lesion. Ultrasound shows a 'doughnut' configuration with hypoechogenic rims and a dense central echogenic core. An urgent surgical opinion should be obtained. If the symptoms have been present for less than 48 hours, and there are no signs of intestinal perforation, a barium or air enema should be given urgently while the surgeon remains nearby. In over 75% of cases it is possible to reduce the intussusception. If the intussusception is not reduced then immediate laparotomy is needed to reduce the lesion manually or to perform an intestinal resection. In about 6% of cases there is a persisting mechanical cause of the intussusception and this will not be detected by the enema.

Inguinal hernia and torsion of testis

Strangulation of an inguinal hernia is likely to be present if the hernia is not reducible easily and there is abdominal pain. Gangrene of an area of small intestine may have already occurred and this part may have to be resected. The danger of strangulation of an inguinal hernia in infants of less than 2 years is considerably greater than at any other time, and any infant with abdominal pain and an inguinal hernia must therefore be admitted for early operation. There is no place for conservative treatment.

The genitalia should be examined in every child with abdominal pain; 25% of cases of testicular torsion present initially with lower abdominal, rather than testicular, pain. A swollen tender testis should be assumed to be a torsion of the testis as orchitis is rare unless the child has mumps. An urgent surgical opinion should be obtained within an hour.

Trauma

If the patient has been in a car crash or had an injury to the abdomen within the previous week the possibility of a ruptured viscus such as the spleen should be considered.

Medical problems

Urinary tract infection

In children with urinary tract infections the pain is usually in one loin but may be central. There may be fever, but dysuria and frequency of micturition are uncommon in younger children. Rarely, haematuria may be present. Microscopy of the urine should be carried out immediately (Figure 8.5) and treatment started if organisms or an excessive number of pus cells are present in the urine (see p. 44).

Henoch–Schönlein purpura

Abdominal pain may precede but usually accompanies the rash and joint swelling of Henoch–Schönlein purpura. The rash, which consists of haemorrhagic papules as well as purpuric spots, appears on the extensor surfaces of the limbs and the buttocks but spares the trunk (Figure 8.6). Blood may be passed rectally.

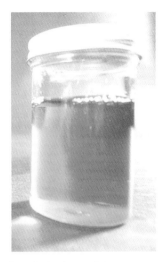

Figure 8.5 Examination of urine is essential.

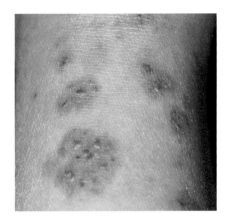

Figure 8.6 Henoch–Schönlein purpura.

Diabetic ketoacidosis

Children with ketoacidosis may have abdominal pain which resolves during treatment with insulin and intravenous fluids. The diagnosis can be excluded by finding a normal blood glucose concentration with a glucometer or by finding no glucose in the urine.

Sickle cell disease

Painful 'crises' occur as a result of occlusion of small blood vessels with distal ischaemia and infarction. Abdominal pain may be caused by occlusion of intestinal or splenic vessels. Other organs commonly affected are the small bones of the hands and feet and the pulmonary vessels. Any child of African or Mediterranean origin who has obscure abdominal pain should have a sickle cell test performed as an emergency and be admitted to hospital (Figure 8.7).

Recurrent abdominal pain of childhood

At least 10% of schoolchildren suffer recurrent abdominal pain, or the periodic syndrome. The condition should be diagnosed

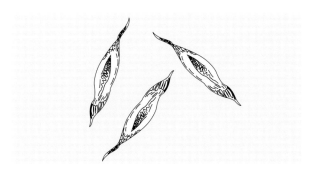

Figure 8.7 Sickle cells.

only in children who have had at least three episodes of pain over longer than 3 months. Two-thirds of the patients have a history of vomiting associated with abdominal pain. There is no abdominal tenderness. The child with recurrent abdominal pain of childhood is just as susceptible as any other child to physical

disease, such as appendicitis. If the pain is present continuously for longer than 6 hours an organic cause must be considered (see Chapter 9).

Gastroenteritis

Gastroenteritis sometimes presents with abdominal pain as the main symptom and is discussed in Chapter 10.

Further reading

Hutson JM, O'Brien M, Woodward AA, Beasely SW. *Jones' Clinical Paediatric Surgery*, 6th edn. Blackwell Publishing, Oxford, 2008.

CHAPTER 9

Recurrent Abdominal Pain

Bernard Valman

Northwick Park Hospital and Imperial College London, UK

OVERVIEW

- Recurrent abdominal pain, which is also called the periodic syndrome, is diagnosed on the basis of at least three episodes of pain in over 3 months.

- At least 10% of schoolchildren have recurrent abdominal pain. The symptoms usually begin at the age of 5 years, although they may appear as early as 2 years or as late as 13 years. In a study of 100 children investigated in hospital only eight were found to have organic causes for the pain, including three with renal problems (Figure 9.1).

- In contrast, 60% of adults with recurrent abdominal pain have a demonstrable physical cause: most have a peptic ulcer, which is uncommon in children, or disease of the biliary tract, which is extremely rare in childhood.

- In children with recurrent abdominal pain the most common emotional state is anxiety and the most common trigger for attacks of pain is events at school.

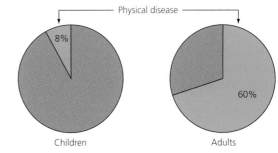

Figure 9.1 Prevalence of physical disease in children and adults with recurrent abdominal pain.

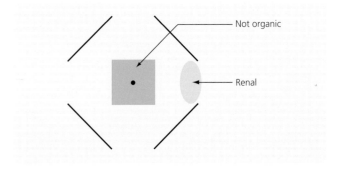

Figure 9.2 Site of pain is an indicator of cause.

History

Details of the first attack may be remembered with special clarity and may help to elucidate the cause. Two-thirds of the children have central abdominal pain, which is usually not organic in origin, but pain in other sites may have a physical cause (Figure 9.2). Pain on one side of the abdomen suggests renal disease. Aggravating and relieving factors should be considered but the type of pain is usually not helpful, and very severe pain causing the child to cry out may still derive from emotional causes. The duration and frequency of the pain, relation to meals, and whether it occurs on a particular day of the week, at weekends, or holidays are all important. Pain that wakes the child at night is likely to have an organic origin.

About two-thirds of the children have vomiting with the pain and 10% have diarrhoea during attacks. Twenty five per cent have headaches and 10% have pain in their limbs between attacks. Pallor during an attack is noticed in half of cases, and one-quarter of children are sleepy after an attack.

If there is a family history of inflammatory bowel disease or peptic ulcer there is an increased risk of these diseases in the child.

Emotional and social factors

In the parents and siblings of children with recurrent abdominal pain the incidence of similar complaints is nearly six times higher than in those of controls. The family member most often affected is the mother. There may be a history of domestic difficulties or parental illness, including depression. Parents should be asked what sort of child their son or daughter is and what disorder they particularly fear in their child. Their reactions to the child should be observed during the visit. The child's attitude to the rest of the family and to friends may need to be explored. The parents must be encouraged to say what they feel, and apparently irrelevant details about everyday life at home and at school may be of diagnostic importance.

ABC of One to Seven, 5th edition. Edited by B. Valman. © 2010 Blackwell Publishing, ISBN: 978-1-4051-8105-1.

Physical disease

Parents as well as doctors are worried about missing physical disease in children with recurrent abdominal pain. A thorough initial clinical examination reassures the parents and should be repeated during an attack if an opportunity arises. For most children all the investigations can be arranged at the first visit and long-term management can be planned.

A specimen of urine should be sent to the laboratory for examination by microscopy and culture from every child with recurrent abdominal pain. Where the pain is having an impact on the life of the child or family, the following additional initial investigations may be performed: full blood count, erythrocyte sedimentaion rate (ESR) and C-reactive protein, renal and liver function tests, and coeliac antibody screen.

Pain in the lateral parts of the abdomen should be investigated by ultrasound examination of the kidneys, bladder, pancreas, and gallbladder (Figure 9.3). The management of upper abdominal pain is controversial, but if the pain does not improve after 2 months of observation it may be necessary to exclude peptic ulcer (by gastroscopy) and chronic pancreatitis (by a radiograph of the abdomen for calcification). If pain is localized to the right hypochondrium ultrasound examination of the gallbladder and liver should be considered.

Recurrent abdominal pain and pronounced weight loss or poor growth suggest the possibility of inflammatory bowel disease or coeliac disease and there may be a raised ESR, raised C-reactive protein, anaemia, high platelet count, or reduced plasma albumin level. Confirmation of inflammatory bowel disease will require endoscopy.

Irritable bowel syndrome is a common cause of recurrent abdominal pain in adults and is being increasingly diagnosed in children. There is no evidence of a structural abnormality and the abdominal discomfort has two out of the following three features:
- Relieved by defaecation;
- Onset associated with change in stool frequency;
- Onset associated with change in form of stool.

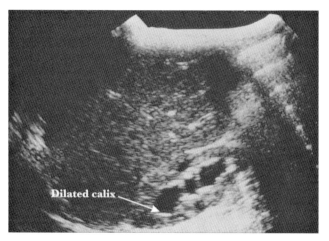

Figure 9.3 Ultrasound examination may show a renal abnormality.

Abdominal distension during episodes of pain may be caused by volvulus with associated malrotation of the gut, and a plain radiograph of the abdomen with the patient erect during an attack is needed. A barium study may help to confirm the diagnosis.

Discussions with child and parents

Ideally, the child should be seen alone, as well as with both parents, at the first visit to explore his feelings about the abdominal pain. At the end of the first interview the most likely diagnosis is discussed with the whole group. If the pain seems to have an emotional origin it is best to explain that a large proportion of children as well as some adults have abdominal pain that has no organic cause but is precipitated by emotional factors. It is important to mention that the child does experience pain, which may be severe, and that he is not pretending. It is helpful to explain that the physical and emotional causes are being explored together and that the child will be reviewed regularly until the pain disappears or has considerably improved. The parents should be asked for their permission for a school report to be requested.

At the second visit it is essential to convince the parents that the likely causes of organic disease have been excluded. The parents may have recollected important details as a result of promptings at the previous visit, or the teacher or family may have discovered a remediable factor at school. The child may be bullied at school, or chance remarks that appear innocuous to a teacher may have a devastating effect on a child. Alternatively, a child may feel very hurt by not being given praise when it is felt to be due. Children are very sensitive to injustice and may treat their teachers as gods. The unreasonable ambition of parents, excessive homework, or going to a large middle school after a small village school may all produce severe stress. Parental discord or separation may be bewildering to a small child. Children who behave superbly in class may show their mother the results of their pent up tension.

With guidance the parents can be shown how to modify the child's environment to help him to adapt. Practical and tactful advice is needed for the inadequate mother who makes excessive emotional demands on her child or for a father who loads the child with his own ambitions. In advising them it is helpful to try to discover why they feel that way. The child cannot be insulated from all stresses, but sources of excessive tension should be removed. If there is frequent absence from school or there is disruption within the family, referral to a child psychiatrist is indicated. Cognitive–behavioural therapy aims to modify thoughts, beliefs, and behavioural responses to symptoms.

Children who have pain every day may need to be admitted to hospital for a short period to take the stress off the family. The object is to determine whether changes in environment will affect the pain, and the opportunity should not be used to carry out an excessive number of investigations. The pain usually abates in hospital, although not always, but may become worse again immediately after the child returns home.

Children with recurrent abdominal pain of emotional origin may also develop physical disease such as acute appendicitis, and if

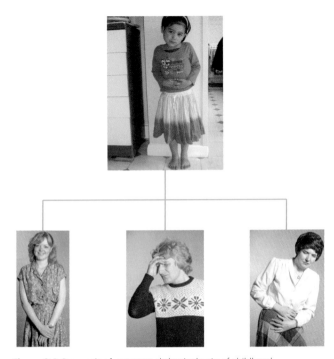

Figure 9.4 Prognosis of recurrent abdominal pain of childhood.

the pain lasts continuously for more than 6 hours the child should be seen again by a doctor as an emergency.

Prognosis

Adolescents and young adults who have attended hospital with recurrent abdominal pain in childhood are later found to have a higher prevalence of continuing symptoms than control subjects (Figure 9.4). These symptoms may consist of continuing attacks of abdominal pain or psychiatric disorders, especially anxiety. Recurrent abdominal pain in childhood may not be as benign as previously believed, but may delineate a group of children who find it difficult to adapt to their environment both as children and as adults.

Further reading

Plunkett A, Beatie RM. Recurrent abdominal pain in childhood. *J R Soc Med* 2005; **98**: 101–106.

CHAPTER 10

Vomiting and Acute Diarrhoea

Bernard Valman

Northwick Park Hospital and Imperial College London, UK

OVERVIEW

- Doctors should always be worried about vomiting in a young child.
- Although it may herald only the onset of a less serious illness, such as acute otitis media, vomiting may be the first symptom of a potentially lethal disease such as meningitis or intestinal obstruction (Box 10.1).
- The child needs to be seen urgently if the vomitus is bile-stained (suggesting intestinal obstruction) or if he is drowsy or refusing feeds, which may occur in meningitis. Diagnosis over the telephone without seeing a vomiting child may be disastrous.
- By the age of 1 year regurgitation of feeds has usually stopped, and vomiting signifies a new illness.

Box 10.1 **Causes of vomiting**

1. Acute gastroenteritis
2. Acute otitis media
3. Periodic syndrome
4. Urinary tract infection
5. Onset of acute appendicitis or intussusception
6. Intestinal obstruction
7. Whooping cough
8. Meningitis
9. Infectious hepatitis

Acute gastroenteritis

Diarrhoea is the passage of loose stools more often than usual. When diarrhoea is severe the stools may be mistaken for urine. When this is a possibility a urine bag should be placed in position and the child nursed on a sheet of polyethylene. Acute gastroenteritis is the most common cause of acute diarrhoea.

Acute gastroenteritis is an acute infection mainly affecting the small intestine, which causes diarrhoea with or without vomiting. In children aged over 3 years abdominal pain may be a prominent feature. The main danger is dehydration and electrolyte imbalance, but the infant may also be very infectious for other infants in a ward or nursery. Gastroenteritis is particularly dangerous to infants aged less than 2 years.

Early signs of dehydration are often difficult to detect, particularly in fat toddlers, but recent weight loss is often a valuable indicator. Sunken eyes, inelastic skin, and a dry tongue are late signs, but if the infant has not passed urine for several hours severe dehydration is probable. The infant must be examined in detail to exclude any other acute infections.

The rotavirus is the most common cause of gastroenteritis in infants and children throughout the world (Figure 10.1). It affects every age group and easily spreads throughout a family, although

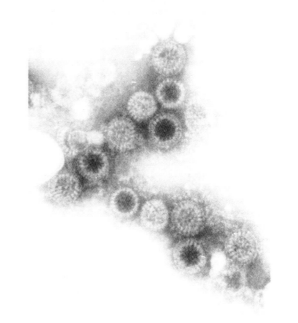

Figure 10.1 Rotavirus.

adults usually have no symptoms but are often carriers of rotavirus. Several distinct episodes of diarrhoea can be caused by the rotavirus as there are several serotypes. The incubation period is 24–48 hours and a respiratory illness, including acute otitis media, precedes the gastrointestinal symptoms in about half of patients. Vomiting which lasts for 1–3 days is followed by abnormal stools for

ABC of One to Seven, 5th edition. Edited by B. Valman. © 2010 Blackwell Publishing, ISBN: 978-1-4051-8105-1.

about 5 days. Treatment is aimed at keeping children well hydrated until they recover spontaneously. The frequency of the stools falls with effective treatment but the consistency of the stools remains abnormal for about a week.

If the patient is given an antibiotic early in the illness subsequent diarrhoea may be attributed to the antibiotic rather than to the rotavirus infection.

Management

Clinical signs of severe dehydration or the loss of 5% or more of body weight are definite indications for admission. If infants relapse after treatment or social problems prevent them being treated at home they may need to be admitted. Infants who vomit persistently usually need to be admitted, although mild symptoms may be managed at home by giving small volumes of liquid by mouth every hour.

In mild cases the main principle of management is to stop cows' milk and solids and give a glucose or sucrose solution orally (Figure 10.2). After 24 hours fruit or vegetable purées may be introduced and then other items from the child's normal diet. Cows' milk and cows' milk products are introduced gradually after the first 24 hours of treatment. Vomiting may be reduced by giving small volumes of fluid frequently. The child should be allowed to drink as much as he wants but needs at least 1 litre each 24 hours.

Kaolin should not be prescribed as it deflects the mother's attention from the main treatment. No antibiotics should be given to children with gastroenteritis treated at home.

The ideal oral rehydrating fluid is a glucose–electrolyte mixture, but a 4% sucrose solution is easily available and safe. Single-dose sachets of glucose–electrolyte powder are available from

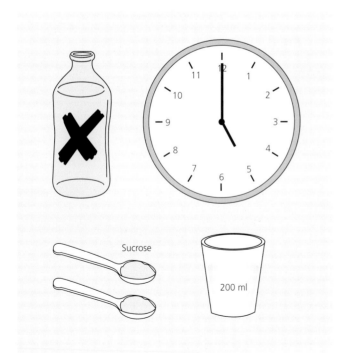

Figure 10.2 Rehydration.

pharmacists without prescription, which enable mothers to make up the mixture accurately at home. A safe alternative is 4% sucrose solution, which can be made up by the mother using 2 level teaspoonfuls of granulated sucrose in 200 mL (6 oz) water. It is dangerous for mothers to add salt to this mixture.

The importance of hand washing and food hygiene should be stressed as spread occurs by the faecal–oral or respiratory routes.

In severe cases of dehydration or persistent vomiting, oral fluids must be replaced with intravenous fluids in infants admitted to hospital (see p. 96). During the next day the fluid requirement should be given as an oral glucose–electrolyte mixture, alternating with full strength cows' milk formula, and fruit and vegetable purées are introduced. Most children are discharged from hospital on normal diets within a few days of admission. Infants in hospital with diarrhoea must be barrier nursed in a cubicle, which should ideally be in an annexe to the children's ward.

Investigations

Ideally, a stool should be sent to the laboratory for detection of pathogens, but this is not necessary for mild cases treated at home. Only a small proportion of children have bacteria such as *Campylobacter*, *Salmonella*, *Shigella*, or pathogenic *Escherichia coli* isolated from their stools. *Cryptosporidium*, a protozoon which can be seen by light microscopy, is a common pathogen. Most cases of gastroenteritis in children are caused by viruses, usually rotavirus, and can be identified by an ELISA slide test. Blood in the fluid stool suggests the presence of Shiga toxin which may cause haemolytic uraemic syndrome.

Children needing intravenous fluids should have their plasma electrolyte, bicarbonate, and urea concentrations measured urgently. If two or more infants in a ward or nursery have diarrhoea at the same time cross-infection should be presumed, even if their stool cultures show no pathogens. Stools from all the infants on the ward should be sent for culture and tested for rotavirus. Admissions to the ward may have to be stopped.

Progress

The infant must be seen again by the doctor within 12 hours of starting treatment to ensure that the illness is resolving, the infant is not losing too much weight, and the mother understands the management. Severe dehydration can occur within a few hours, and it is helpful to have a specific policy to ensure adequate follow-up visits.

The main cause of relapse or persistent symptoms is failure to follow a plan of treatment. Social problems may indicate the need for admission to hospital. A few infants aged less than 2 years have temporary mucosal damage. This causes the diarrhoea to persist for longer than 2 weeks and is considered in Chapter 11.

Gastroenteritis in developing countries

In developing countries the continuation of breastfeeding may be essential for survival. Although infants who are completely breast-fed rarely have severe gastroenteritis, weaning foods made up with

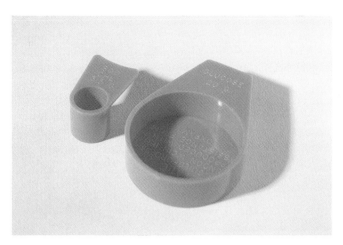

Figure 10.3 Spoons for measuring salt and glucose.

contaminated water may infect a breastfed infant. These infants can be managed by continuing the breastfeeding and supplementing the fluid intake to prevent dehydration until the infant spontaneously recovers. Supplements may be given by mouth in mild cases and intravenously in severe cases. An easier method is to give them by continuous intragastric infusion, for which the fluid does not have to be sterile.

Oral rehydrating fluids can be made up using specially designed spoons to measure the sugar and salt (Figure 10.3). Mothers and older siblings can be taught to use this mixture at the beginning of an episode of diarrhoea rather than wait until the child is dehydrated. Simple slogans such as 'a cup of fluid for every stool' are effective.

Whooping cough

Vomiting may be so severe in infants with whooping cough that the mother is more worried by the vomiting than the cough. During the first 1 or 2 weeks of the illness (catarrhal phase) there is a short, dry, nocturnal cough. Later, bouts of 10–20 short coughs occur both day and night. The cough is dry and each cough is on the same high note or goes up in a musical scale. Vomiting may occur towards the end of a long attack of coughing. The coughing is followed by a sharp indrawing of breath, which causes the whoop. Some children with proved pertussis infection never develop the whoop. Feeding often provokes a spasm of coughing, which may culminate in vomiting. Afterwards there is a short period when the child can be fed again without provoking more coughing. In uncomplicated cases there are no abnormal signs in the respiratory system.

Whooping cough may occur in children who have been fully immunized against it. *Bordetella pertussis* may be isolated from a per nasal swab, which should be plated on a special culture medium immediately after being taken. When the cough has been present for more than a week the culture is usually negative. A blood lymphocyte count of over 10×10^9/L with a normal erythrocyte sedimentation rate suggests whooping cough. A 7-day course of oral erythromycin (or another macrolide) or amoxicillin reduces the infectivity of the patient but does not usually affect the course of the disease if vomiting has already started. Symptomatic treatment

with promethazine or salbutamol to try to reduce the cough usually has little effect, and the parents can be consoled only by being told that the vomiting will eventually stop.

If there are abnormal signs in the respiratory system, the child becomes generally ill, or the cough does not improve after 6 weeks, a chest radiograph is necessary to exclude the secondary complications of bronchopneumonia or lobar collapse, which need treatment with physiotherapy and antibiotics. If the coughing attacks are severe admission to hospital may be necessary. Ideally, the child should be admitted with the mother to an isolation room on the children's ward.

Meningitis

In children aged less than 3 years it is difficult to recognize early signs of meningitis. There may be fever, vomiting, irritability, a high pitched cry, and convulsions. Refusal of feeds and drowsiness are ominous signs. Neck stiffness may be difficult to detect or may be absent.

Older children may have fever, vomiting, and severe headache, but irritability, drowsiness, and unusual behaviour are more useful features. To detect neck stiffness the degree of flexion of the neck is observed when the child is asked to look at his umbilicus. If there is any doubt an attempt can be made to flex the head gently. A test for older children is Kernig's sign, which is present if there is pronounced resistance to extension of the knee when the patient is supine with both the thigh and knee flexed.

A purpuric rash or a discrete maculopapular rash suggests meningococcal infection, and an immediate intravenous or intramuscular injection of benzylpenicillin is needed (Figures 10.4 and 10.5).

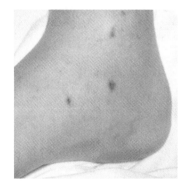

Figure 10.4 Purpuric rash of meningococcal disease.

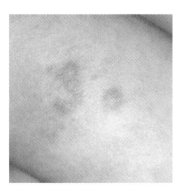

Figure 10.5 Macular rash of meningococcal disease.

The dose is 1200 mg for children over 10 years, 600 mg for children aged 1–9 years, and 300 mg for those under 1 year.

The highest incidence of meningitis occurs between 6 and 12 months of age and the younger the child the more difficult the diagnosis. Lumbar puncture is usually a safe procedure, but herniation of the brainstem and cerebellar tonsils through the foramen magnum can occur if the intracranial pressure is raised appreciably. Although lumbar puncture is the only method of confirming the diagnosis, blood culture will show the causative organism in 70–80% of patients. Indicators of appreciably raised intracranial pressure include papilloedema (which is unreliable), rapidly declining level of consciousness, cranial nerve palsies, and bradycardia. If there is a suspicion of meningococcal disease or appreciably raised intracranial pressure or the infant is shocked, he should be admitted to the intensive care unit, have blood cultures taken, be resuscitated with fluids, and be given antibiotics – and lumbar puncture should be postponed. Every child with meningitis needs intravenous fluids and antibiotics given by bolus injection into the infusion line. Ceftriaxone is the initial drug given to children over 3 months old infected with any of the causative bacteria; the antibiotic may be changed when the antibiotic sensitivity of the pathogen is known.

Further reading

Elliott EJ. Acute gastroenteritis in children. *BMJ* 2007; **334**: 35–40.

CHAPTER 11

Chronic Diarrhoea

Bernard Valman

Northwick Park Hospital and Imperial College London, UK

OVERVIEW

- Diarrhoea that lasts longer than 2 weeks can be called chronic. To provide perspective, diarrhoea starting at any age will be discussed here.

- In the UK, chronic diarrhoea with normal growth between the ages of 1 and 3 years is usually of no sinister significance. It is popularly known as 'toddler diarrhoea' and may be caused by failure to chew food or, alternatively, an excessive intake of drinks containing carbohydrate.

- In developing countries, chronic diarrhoea is often caused by acute or chronic intestinal infection.

- In all parts of the world, acute gastroenteritis may be followed by chronic diarrhoea, and cows' milk protein intolerance and secondary lactase deficiency are contributory causes of this syndrome.

- Malabsorption may be presumed if there is chronic diarrhoea and the growth chart shows inadequate weight gain.

- Coeliac disease and cystic fibrosis are both uncommon; each produces symptoms in about 1 in 2000 children. Inflammatory bowel disease is rare below the age of 7 years.

History and examination

The history should include an enquiry about the duration of the symptoms; the frequency, consistency, and colour of the stools; and whether any fluid is present with the stools. The date when the first gluten was eaten and the detailed diet of an average day need to be recorded. The presence of recognizable foods such as beans, peas, or carrots in the stool is noted. Details of medicines and diets prescribed should be considered.

There are usually few abnormal signs. Abdominal distension and wasting, particularly of the inner aspects of the thighs and of the buttocks, should be noted.

Investigations in children aged over 1 year who have normal growth

Measuring growth as shown on a growth chart is the most valuable single investigation. The chart can often be completed from measurements already recorded in the parent-held record. If growth is normal then severe malabsorption from coeliac disease or cystic fibrosis is unlikely. A normal growth chart and the presence of recognizable food in the stools suggest that the child has toddler diarrhoea (Figures 11.1 and 11.2). This is probably a result of failure

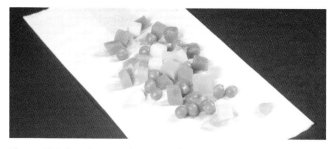

Figure 11.1 Peas, beans, and carrots in the stool suggests toddler's diarrhoea.

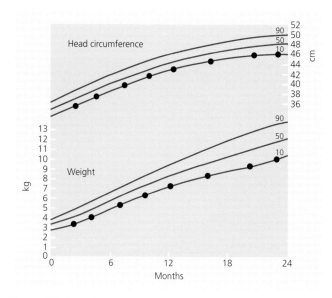

Figure 11.2 Normal growth.

ABC of One to Seven, 5th edition. Edited by B. Valman. © 2010 Blackwell Publishing, ISBN: 978-1-4051-8105-1.

to chew well and will resolve spontaneously. If the intake of drinks containing carbohydrate is excessive, it should be reduced. Apart from examining the stools for pathogens, including *Giardia*, repeat measurements of growth are the only investigation required.

If no recognizable food is present in the stools then cows' milk protein intolerance should be considered (see below).

Investigations in children under 1 year or with poor weight gain

In the UK, cows' milk protein intolerance is the most common cause of chronic diarrhoea in infants under 1 year, in children with poor weight gain, and in children over 1 year with no recognizable food in the stools. The standard guidelines should be followed for investigating each child to avoid missing a rare cause which has a specific treatment (Figure 11.3).

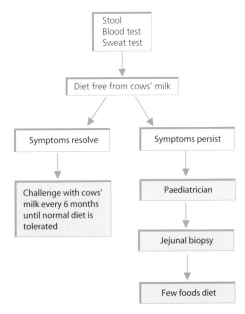

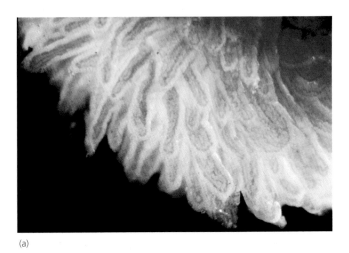

Figure 11.3 Investigations under 1 year or with poor weight gain.

The stools should be examined for parasites including *Giardia*, *Cryptosporidium*, and rotavirus and cultured for pathogens. Blood is taken for a full blood count, erythrocyte sedimentation rate, and estimation of plasma albumin concentration. Screening for coeliac disease is performed by a blood screening test. A sweat test is performed. If all these results are normal, a diet excluding cows' milk and cows' milk products is given for 1 month and supervised by a paediatric dietitian (see below). The dietitian will advise on which proprietary preparation of cows' milk substitute is used locally and will ensure that the calorie, vitamin, and mineral intake are optimal.

Less common causes of chronic diarrhoea

If the blood screening test for coeliac disease is positive, jejunal biopsy is considered. The biopsy is performed through an endoscope with a general anaesthetic or sedation as a day case. A completely flat mucosa on biopsy, devoid of villi, suggests that the child has coeliac disease (Figures 11.4 and 11.5). Similar abnormalities may be found in a wide variety of problems, including gastroenteritis, iron deficiency anaemia, malnutrition, and cows' milk protein intolerance. In these conditions the lesion may be patchy so that a single biopsy may fail to show an abnormal area. See below for management of coeliac disease.

Cows' milk protein intolerance

The prevalence of intolerance to cows' milk protein varies widely according to different workers but is probably about 1 in 100 infants. Diarrhoea starts between birth and 24 months. The intolerance usually resolves by the age of 2 years but may persist until the age of 5 years. Although many abnormalities have been described in laboratory tests none of the tests are easily available or reliable for routine clinical care. The diagnosis depends on withdrawing all products containing cows' milk and challenging the infant with 5 mL boiled cows' milk while under supervision in a day-care unit. If diarrhoea occurs within 24 hours the diagnosis is confirmed and

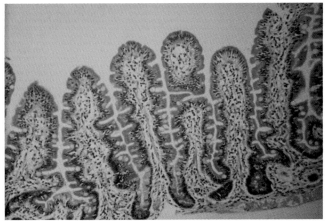

(a)   (b)

Figure 11.4 (a) Scanning microscopic appearance of normal villi. (b) Microscopic appearance of normal villi.

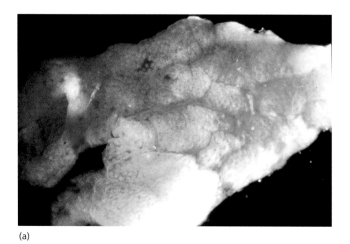

(a)

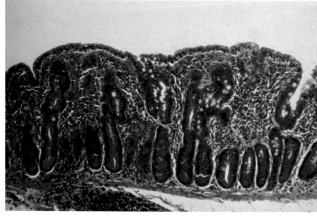

(b)

Figure 11.5 (a) Scanning microscopic appearance of flat mucosa in coeliac disease. (b) Microscopic appearance of mucosa in coeliac disease.

a diet free from cows' milk supervised by a dietitian is prescribed. Some clinicians are prepared to accept the diagnosis if there is a history of recurrent diarrhoea after drinking cows' milk preparations. Affected infants may be given a milk substitute based on milk protein hydrolysate, peptides, or amino acids. Most of these preparations have an unpleasant taste and should be introduced gradually over a week; a soy-based preparation has been used, although up to half of these children eventually become intolerant of it.

If the diarrhoea stops with this diet, a challenge with 5 mL boiled cows' milk is given 6 months later and the volume of milk is doubled each day. If diarrhoea recurs then a diet can be given that contains the volume of milk that previously did not cause diarrhoea. Processed milk in yoghurt or cheese can be tolerated by some children at this stage. If the child has diarrhoea as soon as milk is given a milk-free diet is started again and the milk challenge is repeated every 6 months until the intolerance has resolved.

Infants with cows' milk protein intolerance may also have secondary lactase deficiency. This must be distinguished from isolated lactase deficiency of genetic origin, which causes diarrhoea after the age of 2–3 years. This type is extremely common in various ethnic groups throughout the world but is not found in white races.

Cystic fibrosis

In the UK, cystic fibrosis is the most common autosomal recessive disease in humans. An abnormal gene is inherited from each parent, who is clinically normal, and the risk of a recurrence in each subsequent pregnancy is 1 in 4. One in 25 people in the UK carry the abnormal gene. In cystic fibrosis there is a defect in the transport of salt and water across cell membranes, which causes the production of thick mucus in the lungs and tubular structures throughout the body.

A high sweat sodium concentration is essential for making the diagnosis. If the infant presents with malabsorption resulting from pancreatic insufficiency then vigorous prophylactic treatment of the lungs can be started at an early age and may prevent or limit the development of chronic lung disease (Figure 11.6). The extent

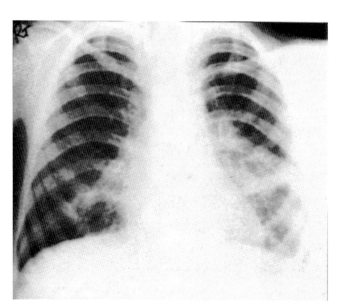

Figure 11.6 Chronic lung disease in cystic fibrosis.

of permanent lung damage determines the ultimate prognosis but the majority of affected children now reach adulthood, probably as a result of more aggressive treatment in the early years. The blood immunoreactive trypsin level is the most reliable neonatal screening test and is now universally available in the UK. Tests for the carrier state and antenatal diagnosis are available for families with one of the detectable gene defects. The most common is Δ508. The steatorrhoea is reduced by giving supplements of pancreatic extract and a diet with a normal fat content. Vitamin supplements are given. Prevention of chronic lung disease depends on regular physiotherapy given by the parents with the liberal use of antibiotics. An oral antibiotic, usually flucloxacillin or erythromycin, is given during every upper respiratory tract infection and during the subsequent 2 weeks. Some authorities give a prophylactic antibiotic continuously during the first year of life. Some children receive antibiotics intravenously or by aerosol at regular intervals to reduce the progression of the lung disease.

Coeliac disease

Coeliac disease is an inflammatory disease caused by sensitivity to the protein gluten, which is found in wheat, rye, and barley. There is a genetic component as there is an increased prevalence in other members of the family.

In coeliac disease malabsorption is associated with a small intestinal mucosa that is flat on diagnosis and improves with a gluten-free diet. Several years may elapse before there is a recurrence of diarrhoea if gluten is reintroduced. The infants present after the age of 5 months but may be seen for the first time at any later age. Some children present after the age of 1 year with chronic diarrhoea but no weight loss. Ideally, the diagnosis should be confirmed by two jejunal biopsies and if it is proved, a gluten-free diet is needed for life. The second biopsy is performed 4–6 months after starting a gluten-free diet and should show an improvement. Especially in children aged under 1 year, a flat jejunal biopsy specimen can be associated with other diseases such as gastroenteritis or cows' milk protein intolerance, and for this reason two biopsies are ideal but may be difficult to achieve. Recent studies suggest that the prevalence of asymptomatic coeliac disease may be as high as 1 in 100 children when whole populations receive the blood screening test.

Specific food intolerance

Ideally, no food should be excluded from a child's diet without a properly controlled observation of symptoms during a period when the child is receiving the suspected food compared with a placebo period. The suspected food should be disguised so that it cannot be distinguished from the placebo by the child. This sophistication is only available at a few centres, but without these facilities overdiagnosis and deprivation of important elements of the diet may occur.

An alternative approach is to give a 'few foods' diet consisting of five or seven specific foods that are known to be least likely to induce diarrhoea in children who are susceptible to intolerance to several foods. Within 2 weeks of starting the diet the diarrhoea stops and a single food is introduced every 3 days until a specific food causes symptoms and can be excluded. In many children no specific cause is found, and the symptoms resolve during the procedure which should last about 6 weeks. This must be supervised by a paediatric dietitian.

Anaphylaxis

Anaphylaxis is an allergic reaction which varies from tingling and swelling of the lips to severe constriction of the airways and sudden fall in blood pressure which may be fatal. It may be caused by an insect sting, for example a bee sting, a drug or a food. There is a greater risk of death if the child has asthma (see p. 24). The foods most commonly involved are peanuts, tree nuts, milk, eggs, fish and shellfish.

A few minutes after exposure there is itching or burning in the lips, mouth, or throat followed by a maculopapular rash with wheals. There may be swelling of the lips, eyelids, tongue, face and neck. Pallor of the skin is followed by drowsiness or loss of consciousness. There may be difficulty with breathing, vomiting, abdominal pain or diarrhoea. An infant may refuse to drink or may dribble.

The airway is secured (see p. 100) and the child is laid flat with the legs raised or on the side if there is a risk of vomiting with aspiration.

Adrenaline is given intramuscularly and repeated every 5 minutes according to the vital signs. Oxygen is given and an intravenous antihistamine such as chlorpheniramine. If there is no improvement, nebulized salbutamol or terbutaline and assisted ventilation may be needed. Intravenous hydrocortisone is given but may take several hours to be effective.

Selected children may be prescribed a syringe with prefilled adrenaline for use in a subsequent emergency at home or at school.

Further reading

Preedy V, Grimble G, Watson R, eds. *Nutrition in the Infant*. Greenwich Medical Media, London, 2001.

Walker WA, Goulet OJ, Kleinman RE, Sherman PM, Shneider BL, Sanderson JR, eds. *Pediatric Gastrointestinal Disease*, 4th edn. BC Decker, Hamilton, Ontario, 2004.

CHAPTER 12

Urinary Tract Infection

Bernard Valman

Northwick Park Hospital, London, UK, and Imperial College London, UK

OVERVIEW

- Each year about two children in each general practice and 300 in each health district have their first urinary tract infection. The ratio of girls to boys affected is about 2:1.

- Identification and treatment of children with infections of the kidneys rather than only the bladder may prevent scarring and some cases of renal failure in adults.

- Vesicoureteric reflux is causally associated with pyelonephritis and renal scarring, which are responsible for 12% of end-stage renal failure in adults.

- Some children with urinary infection have surgically correctable abnormalities such as obstructive lesions or renal stones.

- If severe renal scarring is present, which is rare, it has usually occurred by the age of 5 years. Therefore, early diagnosis and effective treatment are especially important in this age group, but the symptoms may be insidious and the interpretation of routine specimens of urine difficult. The careful collection, handling, and examination of urine specimens is crucial in avoiding unnecessary investigations.

Background

Some adults with hypertension or renal failure have renal scarring (Figure 12.1). Evidence is not yet available to determine whether these scars are caused by a congenital renal abnormality, renal dysplasia, or the result of progressive scarring of the kidneys from recurrent infections in the presence of vesicoureteric reflux. Prompt or prophylactic treatment may prevent the initiation or progression of these scars. Vesicoureteric reflux occurs in 30% of babies whose close relatives have vesicoureteric reflux and in most children resolves by the age of 5 years. The combination of reflux and infection is considered to cause the scarring, although the exact risk is not known. Most scars are present when imaging is first performed, which suggests that the younger infants are most vulnerable – a period when symptoms may be non-specific and urine collection difficult.

ABC of One to Seven, 5th edition. Edited by B. Valman. © 2010 Blackwell Publishing, ISBN: 978-1-4051-8105-1.

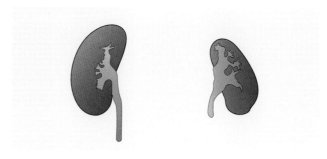

Figure 12.1 Scarring of left kidney.

Clinical features

There may be lethargy, fever, abdominal pain, vomiting, poor feeding, frequency, dysuria, or bed-wetting, but sometimes only fever. The non-specific features are especially common in children aged less than 2 years, who have the highest risk of progressive renal scarring. Only about 20% of children with dysuria and frequency have a urinary infection. Girls with these symptoms often have vulvovaginitis (see p. 150). Children of both sexes may have symptoms due to urate crystals caused by dehydration from deficient fluid intake. Frequency of micturition may be a result of a behaviour problem rather than a urinary tract infection.

As the symptoms are not specific, every ill child without a diagnosis as well as those with the features above must have a properly collected urine specimen examined. This specimen must be taken before any antibiotics are given, and if the child is not dangerously ill it is preferable to withhold antibiotics until a specimen can be examined in the laboratory.

As most scars are present at the first investigation, early diagnosis and prompt treatment are especially important during the first year of life. At home, any infant with a temperature of 38.0°C or above with no definite cause should have a urine sample collected before antibiotics are started. All infants and children admitted to hospital with fever, even with another diagnosis, should have a urine sample taken for examination. The urine should be routinely tested for glucose with a dipstix, but the presence of protein does not confirm a urinary tract infection or its absence exclude it.

Immediate management

Infants younger than 3 months with a possible urinary infection should be referred immediately to the care of a paediatric specialist. Infants and children older than 3 months with evidence of acute pyelonephritis should be admitted to hospital as intravenous antibiotics may be needed. Features of acute pyelonephritis include those of severe illness (see p. 94), fever, abdominal pain, and loin tenderness.

Collection of urine

A clean catch urine specimen from an infant or a mid-stream urine specimen from an older child is the ideal. Only social cleanliness and dryness are required. If these methods are not effective, special urine collecting pads can be used. In infants under 1 year old, if these techniques are not effective, a specimen can be obtained by suprapubic puncture, under ultrasound guidance, or rarely by a catheter specimen in hospital. The collection of urine specimens can be facilitated by a specialist nurse working with general practitioners in the community or open access to a paediatric daycare unit.

Treatment should not be delayed if it is not possible to obtain a sample in a child who is at risk of serious illness.

Specimen transport

The specimen of urine should ideally be collected in a sterile container, cooled immediately to 4°C, and examined in the laboratory within 2 hours. The method and time of collection must be stated on the pathology request to enable the microbiologist to give an accurate opinion. An alternative is to refrigerate the specimen at 4°C in the main compartment of a domestic refrigerator for at most 48 hours before examination. The temperature of the general practice refrigerator should be checked regularly. Another possibility is to transport the urine in 1.8% boric acid, but the correct amount of urine must be added to the bottle to ensure the correct concentration of boric acid.

Criteria for diagnosis of urinary tract infection

Clinical criteria should be used for making a diagnosis when urine testing does not support clinical findings.

Urgent microscopy and culture of the specimen is needed in infants and children younger than 3 years, in those with features of pyelonephritis, and where there is a high or intermediate risk of severe illness (see p. 103). The specimen should be examined before sending it to the laboratory using a dipstix. A positive result for leucocyte esterase and nitrite provides an immediate confirmation that a urinary infection is present but does not provide the antibiotic sensitivities of the pathogen. A negative nitrite test does not exclude a urinary infection as the sensitivity is only 50%. For this reason all urine specimens should be examined by microscopy and culture, but urgent microscopy is only performed with the indications above.

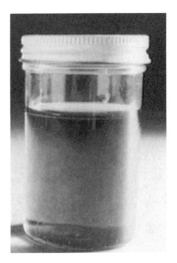

Figure 12.2 Microscopy of urine.

In a child over the age of 3 years who is not acutely ill and has non-specific symptoms, provided the dipstix is negative, a prescription for an antibiotic can be given and started if the diagnosis is confirmed by the laboratory. For all the other groups noted above, an antibiotic is started as soon as a urine specimen has been taken. When the laboratory results have been received the parents should be informed and given advice on prevention and further management.

The diagnosis of urinary infection is confirmed if one specimen yields a pure bacterial growth of more than 100×10^6/L (Figure 12.2). Lower counts of bacteria may be found persistently in urinary infection, particularly in boys. This will be an indication for repeating the culture or obtaining a specimen by suprapubic aspiration. Pyuria (more than 10×10^6/L white blood cells in uncentrifuged urine) is usually found in patients with acute symptoms but is not diagnostic. Pus cells suggest inflammation and may be a helpful indicator in the absence of genital inflammation or when antibiotics have already been prescribed. The absence of pus cells or the presence of a mixed growth of bacteria does not exclude an infection. A urinary infection can only be ruled out if a urine specimen taken before treatment is sterile on culture. Any growth on culture of a catheter or suprapubic specimen is clinically important.

Urine microscopy can make a useful contribution to diagnosis, especially when urgent treatment must be started without awaiting culture results. It has an acceptably low false negative rate and the technique is easily learnt.

Antibacterial treatment

In children with acute symptoms, especially those aged under 3 years, treatment should be started immediately after an appropriate specimen of urine has been obtained. The treatment can be changed after 48 hours when drug sensitivities of the organism are available (Figure 12.3). Trimethoprim is the drug of choice, but the alternative is a cephalosporin. The standard dose is given for 7 days. Prophylactic drugs at a low nightly dose are considered if there has been a previous proved infection. Nitrofurantoin is an additional drug which is useful in prophylaxis, but the high incidence of vomiting makes it unsuitable for the acute phase.

Intravenous antibiotics should be considered if there are features of pyelonephritis.

In children with minor symptoms it is acceptable to wait for the results of the urine culture (which may need to be repeated) before starting treatment.

The urine should be cultured 10 days after the start of treatment, or after 3 days if there is a persistence of symptoms, to check whether the infection has been eliminated or the organism is resistant to the prescribed antibiotic.

A high fluid intake will dilute the urinary bacterial count, stimulate frequent voiding, and ease dysuria.

Detailed discussion with the parents and child is supplemented by written guidelines (Boxes 12.1 and 12.2).

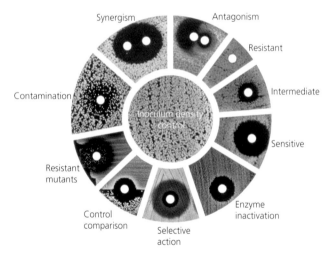

Figure 12.3 Antibiotic sensitivity tests for bacteria.

Box 12.1 **General measures to reduce the risk of recurrent infection and genital soreness in girls**

- Encourage regular bladder emptying 4 hourly or before each meal and before going to bed
- To make sure that the bladder is completely empty ask your child to try again after 5–10 minutes
- Treat constipation adequately with diet and laxatives
- Bath regularly, dry carefully afterwards
- Avoid highly scented soap, do not use bubble bath or wash hair in the bath
- Wipe bottom clean from front to back
- Use soft, absorbent toilet paper
- Ensure easy access to satisfactory toilets at school

Box 12.2 **Information for parents of children with urinary tract infections**

When to suspect urinary tract infection in a child or baby
In a baby or toddler you should think of urinary infection if your child is unwell and has a high temperature, unless there is clear evidence for some other explanation. You should also think of it in a baby who has repeated bouts of fever, vomiting, jaundice, or poor weight gain, and of course in any child who has symptoms related to passing urine.

What to do if you think your child might have a urine infection
It is important to treat urinary tract infection quickly, particularly in very young children, because prolonged infection may make them quite ill and delay in treatment may damage the kidneys. You should contact your doctor as soon as you suspect that your baby or child might have infected urine and ask for an urgent urine test and appointment.

How to diagnose urinary tract infection
Urinary infection can only be diagnosed with certainty if a clean urine sample is collected in a sterile container and sent without delay to the laboratory for examination. The full result will not be available for 48 hours but an immediate indication of the likely result may be obtained from the dipstix test.

Treatment
In babies and toddlers who are unwell and any child with distressing symptoms, your doctor will not wait for the laboratory results but will start treatment straight away with an antibiotic, most commonly trimethoprim. It may be necessary to change the antibiotic after 48 hours if the child is not obviously better. In this case the laboratory result will probably show that the germ causing the infection is not sensitive to the antibiotic first chosen, and will also indicate which other antibiotic to choose. Treatment should be continued for 5–10 days.

What to expect after treatment
Some children who have had a urinary tract infection should have simple tests to check that the kidneys and bladder are normal. If any abnormality is found suitable tests will be arranged. For children the tests may include an ultrasound scan of the kidneys (like the scans used to measure the baby during pregnancy). Further tests will be necessary in very young children and when the ultrasound scan is abnormal. Older children with recurrent distressing symptoms may also need further tests. When the tests have been completed, make sure that you understand the results and the reason why further tests and treatment may be necessary.

What may happen in the future
Boys rarely get further infections, and if they do it usually happens quite soon after the first one. However, girls often do get further infections. It does not necessarily mean that there is something seriously wrong, but it might be an indication for further investigation and a new treatment plan. In some children, long-term, low dose antibiotic treatment is used to reduce the risk of further infections, particularly in very young children who may have some abnormality of the urinary tract (such as vesicoureteric reflux). Ask enough questions so that you understand the reasons for your child's need for prolonged treatment and can help your child to get better.

Adapted from a pamphlet produced by Katherine Verrier Jones, consultant paediatric nephrologist, Royal Infirmary, Cardiff.

Imaging

Recent recommendations have reduced the indications for imaging which have become more selective (Tables 12.1–12.4). Ultrasound examination shows obstructive lesions (Figure 12.4) and large scars, DMSA (^{90m}Tc dimercaptosuccinic acid) isotope scanning detects small scars (Figure 12.5), and cystourethrography detects vesicoureteric reflux (Figure 12.6). It should be performed on the second of a 3-day course of a prophylactic antibiotic.

Follow-up

Repeat urine microscopy and culture is advisable at times of fever or recurrence of symptoms. Where scars have been detected, the child's growth and blood pressure should be measured regularly.

If an anatomical abnormality is detected radiologically or if infection recurs the radiological investigations may need to be repeated to assess whether renal growth is normal and whether there is evidence of fresh scarring. The intervals between these

Table 12.1 Imaging tests: definitions.

Atypical UTI	Recurrent UTI
• Seriously ill (see Chapter 27) • Poor urine flow • Abdominal or bladder mass • Raised creatinine • Septicaemia • Failure to respond to treatment with suitable antibiotics within 48 hours • Infection with non-*E. coli* organisms	• Two or more episodes of UTI with acute pyelonephritis/upper urinary tract infection • One episode of UTI with acute pyelonephritis/upper urinary tract infection plus one or more episode of UTI with cystitis/lower urinary tract infection • Three or more episodes of UTI with cystitis/lower urinary tract infection

Table 12.2 Recommended imaging schedule for infants younger than 6 months.

Test	Responds well to treatment within 48 hours	Atypical UTI*	Recurrent UTI*
Ultrasound during the acute infection	No	Yes[‡]	Yes
Ultrasound within 6 weeks	Yes[†]	No	No
DMSA 4–6 months following the acute infection	No	Yes	Yes
MCUG	No	Yes	Yes

*See Table 12.1 for definitions.
[†]If abnormal consider MCUG.
[‡]In an infant or child with a non-*E. Coli*-UTI, responding well to antibiotics and with no other features of atypical infection, the ultrasound can be requested on a non-urgent basis to take place within 6 weeks.

Table 12.3 Recommended imaging schedule for infants and children older than 6 months but younger than 3 years.

Test	Responds well to treatment within 48 hours	Atypical UTI*	Recurrent UTI*
Ultrasound during the acute infection	No	Yes[‡]	No
Ultrasound within 6 weeks	No	No	Yes
DMSA 4–6 months following the acute infection	No	Yes	Yes
MCUG	No	No[†]	No[†]

*See Table 12.1 for definitions.
[†]While MCUG should not be performed routinely it should be considered if the following features are present:
• dilatation on ultrasound
• poor urine flow
• non-*E. coli*-infection
• family history of VUR.
[‡]In an infant or child with a non-*E. Coli*-UTI, responding well to antibiotics and with no other features of atypical infection, the ultrasound can be requested on a non-urgent basis to take place within 6 weeks.

Table 12.4 Recommended imaging schedule for children 3 years or older.

Test	Responds well to treatment within 48 hours	Atypical UTI*	Recurrent UTI*
Ultrasound during the acute infection	No	Yes[†‡]	No
Ultrasound within 6 weeks	No	No	Yes[†]
DMSA 4–6 months following the acute infection	No	No	Yes
MCUG	No	No	No

*See Table 12.1 for definitions.
[†]Ultrasound in toilet-trained children should be performed with a full bladder with an estimate of bladder volume before and after micturition.
[‡]In a child with a non-*E. Coli*-UTI, responding well to antibiotics and with no other features of atypical infection, the ultrasound can be requested on a non-urgent basis to take place within 6 weeks.

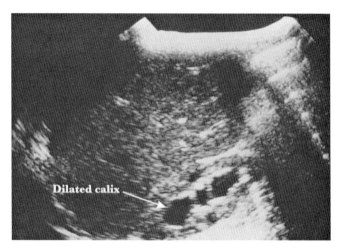

Figure 12.4 Ultrasound of kidneys showing dilated calyx.

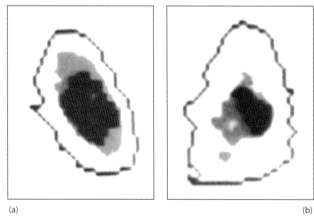

(a)　　　　　　　　　　　　　　　　(b)

Figure 12.5 DMSA scan: (a) normal; (b) abnormal.

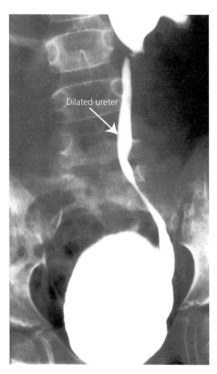

Figure 12.6 Micturating cystogram.

investigations vary with the problem, and excessive radiation can be avoided by consulting a paediatrician.

Continuous prophylaxis

The object of prophylaxis is to prevent reinfection of a susceptible urinary tract after bacteriuria has been eliminated. Prophylaxis should be considered in children with vesicoureteric reflux, those with recurrent symptomatic infection, and children with renal damage. The ideal drug should be absorbed high in the alimentary tract, be excreted in high concentration in the urine, and not cause resistance in the flora of the lower bowel. Trimethoprim and nitrofurantoin fulfil these criteria, and a single daily dose of about half the standard 24-hour dose should be given in the evening. Nitrofurantoin has the disadvantage that it often causes nausea and vomiting even at this low dose. These patients are best managed at a special urinary tract infection clinic at the local district hospital.

Further reading

Coultard MG. Is reflux nephropathy preventable, and will the NICE UTI guidelines help? *Arch Dis Child* 2008; **93**: 196–200.
National Institute for Clinical Excellence (NICE). *Urinary Tract Infection in Children; Diagnosis, Treatment and Long-Term Management.* NICE Clinical Guideline 54, 2007.

CHAPTER 13

Nocturnal Enuresis

Bernard Valman

Northwick Park Hospital and Imperial College London, UK

OVERVIEW

- Wetting the bed is normal at birth, a nuisance at 5 years, and then it becomes increasingly disturbing for child and parents. Siblings who share the same room or bed and the family whose living room is dominated by wet sheets resent the problem.

- Ten per cent of children still wet the bed at the age of 5 and 14% of these become dry each succeeding year (Figure 13.1).

- A physical cause should be excluded in those who are wet during the day as well as at night.

- The electric enuresis alarm (buzzer) is an effective aid but an enthusiastic teacher of the use of the alarm contributes to its success.

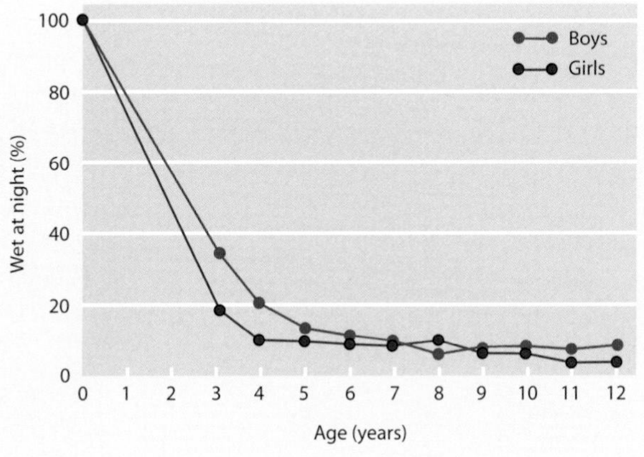

Figure 13.1 Percentage of children wet at night related to age.

History

The mother should be asked for the longest period that the child has been dry at night. If the child has been dry for at least two nights in succession there is likely to be no structural abnormality of the renal tract. If the enuresis started after a long period of dryness (secondary enuresis) a precipitating event should be sought. Common precipitating factors are the birth of a brother or sister, marital discord, admission to hospital, maternal illness, or moving home.

A urinary tract infection may cause frequency of micturition and enuresis and should be excluded in every child with enuresis.

Ten per cent of children with nocturnal enuresis also wet themselves during the day, and a distended bladder or a spinal lesion should be considered. Poor stream in boys suggests an abnormality of the urinary tract. A neurological abnormality severe enough to cause bladder problems will usually interfere with walking.

The reason for referral at a particular time rather than earlier may indicate the need for treatment. The child may be motivated to change – for example, because he wants to go to a camp.

Enuresis to a late age in one of the parents suggests a familial pattern of delayed maturation. Delay in other aspects of development may show that the child has other abnormalities.

Examination

Enlarged kidneys or bladder and midline naevi or other markers of spinal abnormality should be sought. The reflexes at the ankles, gait, and sensation over the sacral area should be examined. In every case a sample of urine must be sent to the laboratory to exclude infection, and glycosuria can be excluded by a dipstix test. Unless there is a specific indication other than enuresis an ultrasound examination of the kidneys should not be performed.

Treatment

No treatment is indicated for a child under the age of 4½ years. Ideally, the parents and child should be seen together at first and then the child separately. The child should be given an opportunity to explain what he feels and to be shown that he is the patient and it is his cooperation that is necessary for success.

Fluid restriction is not helpful. Charts with stars provide a method whereby the child keeps records (Figure 13.2). Young children enjoy filling the spaces, and the recording of dry nights should be emphasized. Some children become completely dry after

ABC of One to Seven, 5th edition. Edited by B. Valman. © 2010 Blackwell Publishing, ISBN: 978-1-4051-8105-1.

using a chart for a few weeks without any other treatment. However, some paediatricians find that this method is very disheartening to the child who is not successful.

Lifting the child on to a potty before the parents go to sleep is sometimes associated with a dry bed in the morning. This treatment can be used until a decision is made to use a buzzer.

Buzzer treatment

Children over the age of 6 use the alarm easily but it can be successful at the age of 5. Whether the child sleeps in his own bed and in his own room will determine whether a standard buzzer can be used. Temporary changes in sleeping arrangements may be necessary to prevent others in the room being woken by the buzzer. A special alarm that vibrates the pillow can be used where sleeping arrangements cannot be changed and for children who do not wake when the buzzer sounds.

Hospitals, health centres, and local health clinics have stocks of alarms, but expert advice on the use of the buzzer is needed from a committed person. This could be a doctor, nurse, or health visitor. The child and mother must be shown how to arrange the alarm in the bed and how to test it.

There are two types of detector, each of which is attached to an alarm. In the first type, a miniature sensor (3 cm in length) is attached to the child's pants and the alarm is attached to the pyjama top near the collar bone (Figure 13.3a). The second type of detector consists of single or paired mats (Figure 13.3b). The child sleeps on a sheet which separates him from a detector – a metal mat – connected to an alarm buzzer. When the child passes urine the circuit is completed. The alarm wakens the child, who stops the urine stream, gets out of bed, turns off the alarm, and goes to the lavatory. The amount of urine passed before the child wakes becomes progressively smaller and he either wakes before the alarm starts or sleeps throughout the night without passing urine. The child should be seen a week after issuing the alarm and then at longer intervals. After he has been dry for 6 consecutive weeks the alarm is removed from the bed but kept at home ready for use, if necessary, for a further 6 weeks. About 80% of the children become dry within 4 months and most within the first 2 months of treatment. About 10% of children relapse but respond quickly to a second course of treatment with the alarm.

Five to 20% of children will still be wetting the bed after 4 months' treatment and these should be given a respite of a year before using the alarm again.

Drugs and psychiatrists

If treatment with an enuresis alarm is not successful then desmopressin tablets or nasal spray can be given at bedtime. It reduces urine production by an antidiuretic effect on the renal tubules. A course of treatment should not exceed 2 months. This treatment has a high success rate which may be similar to the results with an alarm. This treatment can be used for special events such as staying at a friend's house or going to camp.

	1st Week	2nd Week	3rd Week	4th Week	
Monday		★		★	
Tuesday			★	★	
Wednesday	★		★	★	
Thursday		★	★	★	
Friday				★	
Saturday		★	★	★	
Sunday	★			★	

Figure 13.2 Star chart.

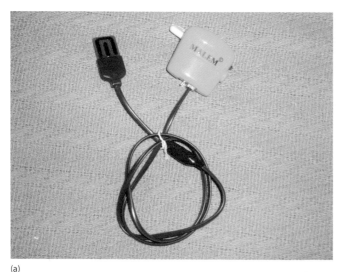

(a)

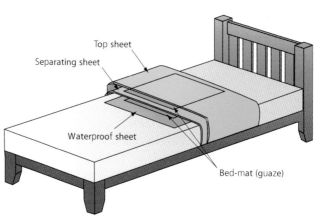

Top sheet
Separating sheet
Waterproof sheet
Bed-mat (guaze)

(b)

Figure 13.3 (a) Miniature sensor, wire and alarm. (b) Mat type of enuresis alarm.

Tricyclic antidepressants have been used successfully in enuresis but there is a high relapse rate when the drug is stopped. A disadvantage of this treatment is that the pleasant-tasting medicine has caused severe side effects and death through children taking overdoses. These drugs are not recommended.

When enuresis is a part of an emotional disorder the child should be referred to a child psychiatrist. Chronic constipation or the passage of formed stools in inappropriate places may occur with enuresis in a severely disturbed child. Enuresis starting after a long period of dry nights suggests a precipitating cause – for example, separation of parents. If buzzer treatment has failed, the possibility of an underlying emotional cause should be sought again.

Further reading

ERIC. Education and resources for improving childhood continence. www.eric.org.uk

CHAPTER 14

Systolic Murmurs

Bernard Valman

Northwick Park Hospital and Imperial College London, UK

OVERVIEW

- Congenital heart disease occurs in about 1 in every 140 live births but the most common clinical problem is the child with a murmur discovered during a routine examination or during an acute illness. Most of these children have no cardiac disease.

- The minority with physical disease usually have a ventricular septal defect. Most of the ventricular septal defects close spontaneously before the child reaches the age of 5 years.

- Loud murmurs are always caused by cardiac disease. Soft murmurs may be either caused by cardiac disease or have no pathological importance (benign or innocent murmurs).

- Every child with a murmur should be referred to a paediatric cardiologist who will examine the child and carry out an echocardiogram to confirm the diagnosis.

Symptoms

Congenital heart disease may present in the neonatal period with slow feeding, a raised respiratory rate, or cyanosis. Slow weight gain and dyspnoea on exertion may be the presenting features in the older infant or child. Some children with congenital heart disease have no symptoms. The most common clinical problem is the infant or child with no symptoms, who is found to have a cardiac murmur during a routine examination or during a minor illness.

Loud systolic murmurs

Ventricular septal defect is the most common congenital heart disease in childhood (Figure 14.1). It produces a loud murmur maximal in the fourth left intercostal space close to the sternum. Although it is maximal at that site it radiates in all directions and may be heard as high as the clavicle.

Pulmonary stenosis causes a loud systolic murmur maximal in the pulmonary area, which is conducted to the left lung posteriorly.

Aortic stenosis produces a murmur that may be maximal to the right of the upper sternum and to the left of the mid-sternum and is well conducted to both sides of the neck.

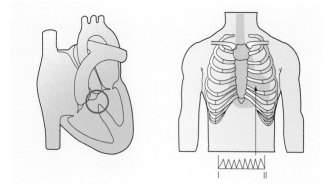

Figure 14.1 Ventricular septal defect.

Soft systolic murmurs caused by organic disease

Atrial septal defect causes a soft systolic murmur in the pulmonary area because of the increased flow of blood through the pulmonary valve. This lesion is often first noted in adult life, when the symptoms appear. In atrial septal defect the second heart sound is widely split and does not vary with respiration. In contrast, in normal children the second heart sound is widely split in inspiration and less in expiration.

Children with coarctation of the aorta often have a short systolic murmur heard over the back between the scapulae. The femoral arteries should be palpated routinely (Figure 14.2). Children with coarctation of the aorta often have other lesions, such as aortic stenosis, and the finding of a murmur resulting from that lesion may bring the coarctation to light.

Differential diagnosis

For those who are not cardiologists, systolic murmurs that spill over into diastole may be difficult to differentiate from purely systolic murmurs. There are two important examples: patent ductus arteriosus and the venous hum. Most children with persistent patent ductus arteriosus have no symptoms (Figure 14.3). The murmur is maximal in the second left intercostal space lateral to the pulmonary area. The murmur may radiate down the left sternal edge and to the apex. The murmur is described as sounding like machinery. The murmur is present when the ductus is widely patent.

ABC of One to Seven, 5th edition. Edited by B. Valman. © 2010 Blackwell Publishing, ISBN: 978-1-4051-8105-1.

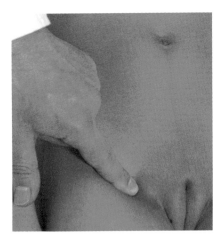

Figure 14.2 Femoral pulse.

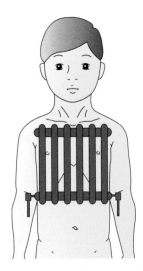

Figure 14.4 Benign murmur corresponds to noisy radiator.

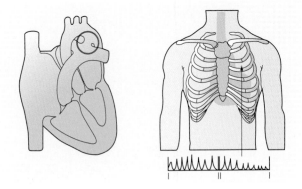

Figure 14.3 Patent ductus arteriosus.

Other types of congenital heart disease, particularly ventricular septal defect, may also be present.

The venous hum is a continuous murmur throughout systole and diastole and is heard best under the inner end of the right clavicle with the child sitting up. It can be abolished by lying the child down. It is a normal finding.

Soft systolic murmurs of benign origin

Benign systolic murmurs are soft, short, and low pitched. They are heard maximally to the left of the sternum. The murmur becomes louder when the patient lies down and softer when standing up. Organic disease is usually excluded by the character of the murmur and the absence of any symptoms or abnormal signs in the cardiovascular system. The femoral pulses must be checked. Echocardiography confirms that the cardiovascular system is normal.

Fever or anaemia intensifies benign murmurs and a murmur that sounded loud at the time of an acute illness may be almost inaudible in an outpatient clinic a few weeks later. Anaemia may be difficult to diagnose clinically and a haemoglobin estimation is advisable.

Benign murmurs: discussion with parents

Benign or innocent murmurs do not indicate heart disease and need no treatment. Many parents fail to understand what the murmur means despite careful explanation and unnecessary fear and anxiety is generated. Despite reassurances by a doctor the parents may restrict the physical activities of the child, to his detriment. The parents may misinterpret what is told to them and believe that their child has heart disease.

If the murmur has been noted on one occasion it is likely to be heard again at routine examinations and whenever the child has a fever. If the child is acutely ill with a high fever, the murmur is louder.

When the murmur is being discussed, preferably in the presence of both parents, it should be emphasized that it is a normal sound heard in children with normal hearts; that the noise is caused by blood flowing through the tubes, and in some cases more noise is produced than in others, similar to the noise in some central heating systems (Figure 14.4). Doctors initially have to exclude disease but when they have done that the child should be considered completely normal and should be treated as a normal child. Ample opportunity must be given to allow the parents to ask questions to enable them to understand this difficult concept.

Further reading

Anderson RH, Baker ES, MaCartney FJ, Rigby Ml, Shinebourne EA, Tynan M, eds. *Paediatric Cardiology*, 2nd edn. Churchill Livingstone, London, 2002.

CHAPTER 15

Growth Failure

Bernard Valman

Northwick Park Hospital and Imperial College London, UK

OVERVIEW

- Parents may be worried because they consider their child to be too short, or too thin, or both.

- Infants' heights are usually not noticed until they start walking and are compared with their contemporaries. This coincides with the period of negativism and a normal reduction in appetite and food intake.

- Most children whose parents seek advice have familial short stature but the rest have a wide variety of problems, some of which can be improved after an accurate diagnosis has been made.

This chapter is concerned mainly with growth after the age of 1 year, but some aspects of earlier growth have been included to put the topic into perspective. Growth is a dynamic process and more than one accurate measurement is needed to assess it. Infants under 1 year are weighed with a napkin in place, but over 1 year children wear vest and pants only. Weight can be measured accurately with minimum skill and cheap equipment. This allows any deviations from normal to be detected within a few weeks during the time of rapid growth – that is, during the first few months of life. Another index is needed for comparison, and until the age of 2 years the head circumference is reliable. After the age of 1 year standing height can be measured, but attention to detail is needed to provide reproducible results. The head must be held with the external auditory meatus and the outer angle of the eye in the same horizontal plane and gentle upward traction applied to the mastoid processes (Figure 15.1). Two measurements 6 months apart must be made before the rate of growth can be assessed confidently.

Too thin or too light

A child is usually on a similar centile for weight, head circumference, and height. Children of tall parents tend to be towards the 98th centile and those of short parents near the 0.4 centile (Figure 15.2). After the age of 2 years most children remain on the same centiles for the

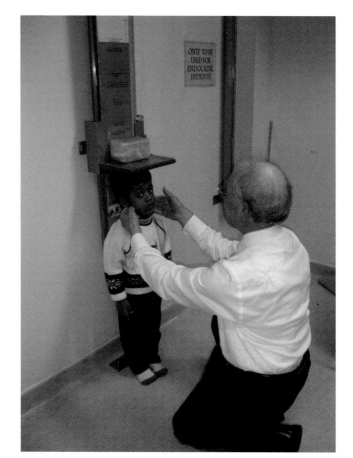

Figure 15.1 Measuring height.

rest of their lives. Plotting these measurements on a chart in routine clinics helps to confirm that the child is receiving adequate food and is growing normally. Although birth weight depends mainly on maternal size, some children are more like one parent than the other in final size (Figure 15.3). By the age of 2 years these adjustments have usually been made. If only their weights are recorded children may seem to be either failing to thrive if the father is small, or gaining weight excessively if the father is tall. If height and head circumference are plotted together the series of measurements can be seen to be parallel.

The child who is abnormally thin has lost subcutaneous fat, which is shown by wasting of the buttocks and the inner aspects

ABC of One to Seven, 5th edition. Edited by B. Valman. © 2010 Blackwell Publishing, ISBN: 978-1-4051-8105-1.

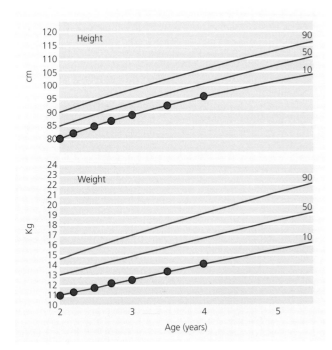

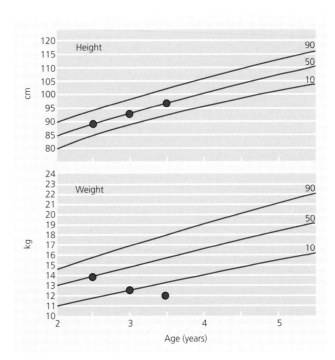

Figure 15.2 Familial short stature.

Figure 15.4 Wasted child.

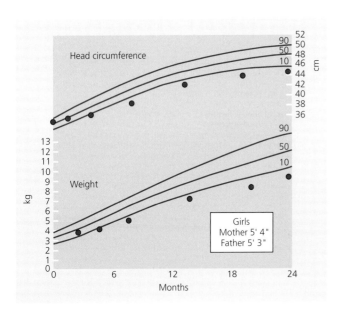

Figure 15.3 Taking after father.

of the thighs. The growth chart then shows a weight that is on a centile considerably lower than that of the head circumference or height (Figure 15.4). A child from a family of a narrow body build may show a similar pattern if measured only once but there will be no clinical signs of wasting, and if the measurements are repeated after an interval the increase in weight will parallel that in height or head circumference.

Familial patterns of growth

Most children have a height about midway between those of their parents when an adjustment for sex has been made (Figure 15.5).

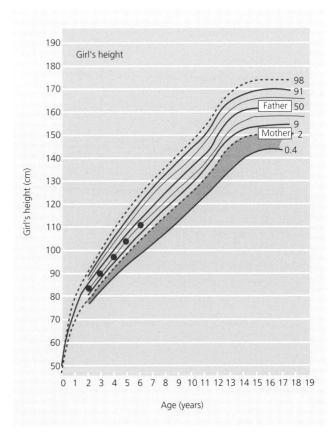

Figure 15.5 Height is midway between parents.

For boys, 12 cm should be added to the sum of the parents' heights and for girls this should be subtracted. Division of this total by two gives the expected adult height for that child. Alternatively, the height centile for each parent can be determined from the chart that ends at 19 years, and the child usually has a centile between the two values.

A child with familial short stature will follow the growth pattern of both or one of the parents or another close relative, but the diagnosis needs to be confirmed by checking that he is growing along or parallel to one of the centile lines This is called normal variant or constitutional short stature.

Normal rate but atypical patterns of growth

Most infants who grow poorly before birth have a period of 'catch up' growth during the first few months of life (Figure 15.6). However, a few continue to grow at the same rate after birth. Although they are short their body proportions are normal but they never reach the normal range for height and weight.

Some short schoolchildren have a family history of similar delay in growth and development, and during the school years the height and bone age are usually retarded. This is called maturational delay. Final height is similar to that expected from the heights of the parents. These children, especially the boys, may become very distressed towards puberty, when they realize that they are not growing as fast as their friends who experience a prepubertal growth spurt before they do. Sympathetic explanation provides a boost to the morale of children with familial maturation delay, but referral to a paediatrician to consider a short course of androgen treatment to accelerate puberty is indicated if there is emotional disturbance.

Deficient food or malabsorption

Malnutrition from lack of food probably occurs in some of the lower socioeconomic classes in affluent countries as well as in developing countries. Unrecognized poor lactation is becoming more prominent as the incidence of breastfeeding increases. Psychosocial deprivation may decrease the amount of food eaten and may be associated with temporary growth hormone deficiency. Cystic fibrosis and coeliac disease are the most common causes of severe malabsorption, although only 1 in 2000 children is affected by each of these diseases (Figures 15.7 and 15.8).

Endocrine problems and other disorders

Children with hypothyroidism may have no distinctive clinical features, and the diagnosis is often delayed. Girls with untreated

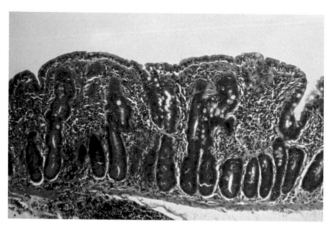

Figure 15.7 Coeliac disease.

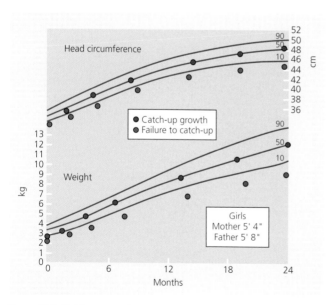

Figure 15.6 Catch-up growth.

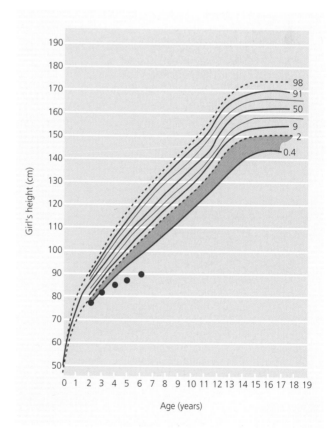

Figure 15.8 Deficient food or malabsorption.

congenital adrenal hyperplasia are virilized. Growth hormone deficiency should be suspected if a child is extremely short and is below the 0.4 line on the height chart or growth is less than 5 cm in a year.

If previous measurements are not available the child should be measured again 6 months later. If the growth curve is not on or parallel to a centile line or the child has grown less than 2.5 cm he should be referred to a paediatrician.

The mechanism whereby children with cerebral palsy, uraemia, chronic heart failure, and liver disease fail to grow well is complex, but most of these children have a poor appetite and are likely to have a deficient food intake.

Infants with obvious bone disease such as achondroplasia, as well as other children with named syndromes, can be recognized by their abnormal appearance and the systems affected. Girls with Turner's syndrome may have no gross abnormalities on physical examination, and leucocyte chromosome studies are needed to exclude this diagnosis.

Referral to hospital

If a child's low height centile is similar to that of a parent or close relative and he has no symptoms or abnormal signs then familial short stature can be diagnosed. This should be confirmed by measuring the child again 6 months later and showing that he is growing on a line that is parallel to the third centile – that is, at a normal rate.

Children with any of the following features should be referred to hospital for further investigation:

1 Clinical signs of wasting.
2 Symptoms such as dyspnoea on exercise or chronic diarrhoea.
3 Abnormal appearance or signs of disease such as congenital heart disease.
4 Documented evidence of a slow rate of growth (less than 2.5 cm) detected by two measurements 6 months apart.
5 Height below the 0.4 centile line on the growth chart.
6 Social problems or deprivation. About one-third of children below the second centile who have no physical disease come from severely deprived backgrounds and are not only stunted physically but also retarded in tests of intellectual function. Some of these children are suffering from neglect.

Patients seen in hospital will have their height and weight measured carefully. A radiograph of the left hand is taken to measure the

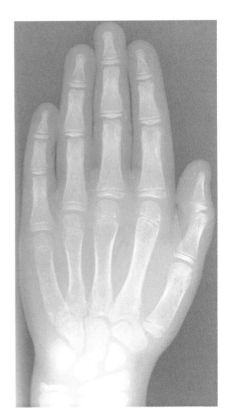

Figure 15.9 Bone age.

bone age (Figure 15.9) and blood is taken to estimate erythrocyte sedimentation rate, haemoglobin, plasma thyroxine, thyrotrophin, albumin, and creatinine concentrations. Girls with documented slow growth have blood taken for chromosomal analysis. A sweat test for cystic fibrosis is performed and blood screening tests for coeliac disease performed. A test for growth hormone secretion after stimulation is performed last because some of the previous conditions may cause confusingly low levels and many paediatricians prefer to estimate the growth rate first.

Further reading

Brook C, Clayton P, Brown R. *Brook's Clinical Paediatric Endocrinology*. Blackwell Publishing, Oxford, 2005.

CHAPTER 16

Prevention and Management of Obesity

Bernard Valman

Northwick Park Hospital and Imperial College London, UK

> **OVERVIEW**
>
> - The prevalence of obesity is increasing in both children and adults. About 10% of schoolchildren are obese.
> - Obese infants and children tend to become obese adults, who may develop diabetes, high blood pressure, heart disease, and arthritis.
> - Treatment to reduce established obesity in children is difficult and often unsuccessful.
> - A planned approach to nutrition should be started at weaning and may be necessary throughout childhood to prevent obesity.

Prevention

Milk has a bland taste because it has low concentrations of sugar, salt, and fat. Weaning foods have a semisolid or solid consistency but also have stronger flavours. The flavour of any food can be improved by adding sugar, salt, or fat, or all three. To make foods attractive and encourage children to eat a larger amount, food manufacturers add these substances to foods and mothers are tempted to follow this lead.

When a baby first receives weaning foods he is usually enthusiastic. As he approaches the age of 12 months his appetite falls and he may take a smaller amount or none of a particular food. The face, trunk, and limbs become thinner because of a reduction in body fat. About this time the infant enters the phase when he is trying to exert his individuality. The mother notices that the infant is becoming thinner as well as refusing food. The infant may be tempted with more tasty food in the mistaken idea that he needs more food to continue to gain weight at the previous rate. These tempting foods often come from the mother's plate and may be high in sugar, salt, and fat. The infant develops a taste for these highly flavoured foods and although he may eat only small quantities, he has developed a dislike for bland foods which will be lifelong and may lead to later obesity. A reduced appetite and becoming thinner at the age of 1 year is normal (Figure 16.1) and offering tempting food is not needed.

Early detection of obesity

If excessive weight gain is suspected, measure the child's height and weight, calculate the body mass index (BMI) and plot it on a BMI chart (Figure 16.1). If the BMI is above the 91st centile, refer the child to a paediatrician or dietitian. There has been a suggestion that all children should have their heights and weights measured once a year and plotted on a BMI chart. This would provide an early warning of excessive weight gain. At present this is not national policy, but parents could make this assessment provided that they have access to BMI charts.

The obese child is tall for his age initially. Puberty develops early and the final height is shorter than would be expected from growth charts. The genitalia of boys may appear small as a result of being buried by fat.

Management of obesity

Obesity is caused by an excessive calorie intake with insufficient exercise. Some families have a strong history of obesity which may represent a genetic factor or a long-standing family custom to eat excessive calories.

There is a causative disease in less than 1% of children with obesity and this causes a reduction in height as well as obesity. If the child is short or has a falling centile for height, has dysmorphic features or learning difficulties the following investigations should be considered:

- Thyroid function;
- 24-hour urinary free cortisol;
- Genetic tests.

Reducing calorie intake

The goal is to reduce the child's weight or to maintain the present weight depending on the age and stage of growth. If the child is growing rapidly in height it may be necessary only to maintain the present weight as the growth in height will ensure that the weight gradually becomes appropriate for the increased height. The diet should be tailored to the child's preferences avoiding hunger. The total energy intake should be reduced below the expenditure by reduction in fat and sugar. Snacks between meals should be avoided (Figure 16.2) and food should not be offered as a reward for attaining a goal. In obese children a weight loss of 450 g (1 lb) per month

ABC of One to Seven, 5th edition. Edited by B. Valman. © 2010 Blackwell Publishing, ISBN: 978-1-4051-8105-1.

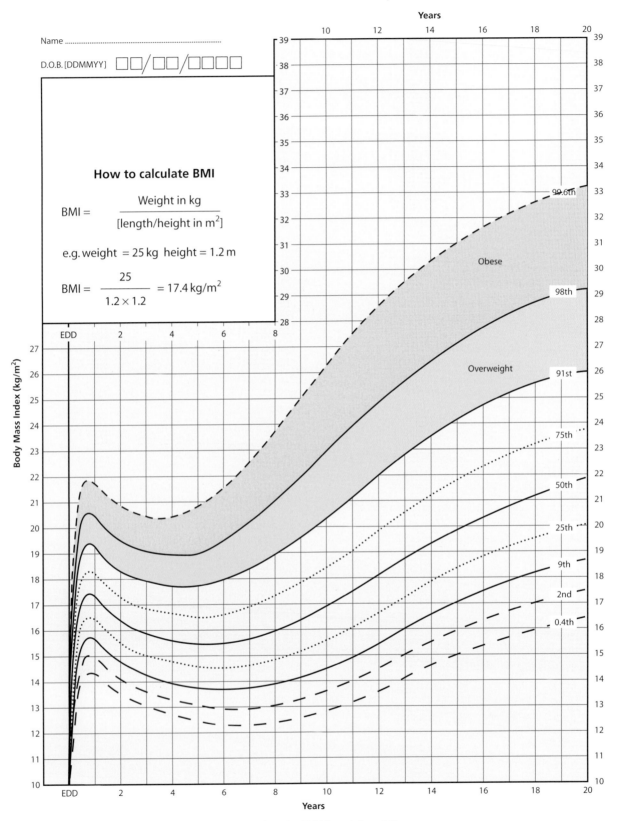

Name ....

D.O.B. [DDMMYY] ☐☐/☐☐/☐☐☐☐

How to calculate BMI

$$BMI = \frac{\text{Weight in kg}}{[\text{length/height in m}^2]}$$

e.g. weight = 25 kg height = 1.2 m

$$BMI = \frac{25}{1.2 \times 1.2} = 17.4 \text{ kg/m}^2$$

Figure 16.1 Body mass index (BMI) chart. Reprinted with permission from the Child Growth Foundation.

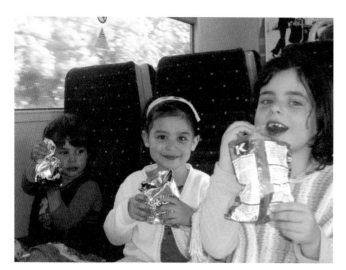

Figure 16.2 Junk food is not healthy.

> Box 16.1 **Healthy diet for the whole family**
>
> - Base meals on starchy foods such as potatoes, bread, rice, and pasta, choosing wholegrain where possible
> - Eat plenty of fibre-rich foods such as oats, beans, peas, lentils, grains, seeds, fruit, and vegetables as well as wholegrain bread, brown rice and pasta
> - Eat at least five portions of a variety of fruit and vegetables a day in place of foods high in fat and calories (two portions for children under 2 years)
> - One portion of a protein food a day (fish, meat, eggs , cheese, or other dairy food)
> - Choose low-fat foods
> - Avoid foods containing a lot of fat and sugar, such as fried food, sweetened drinks, sweets, and chocolate. Some takeaways and fast foods contain a lot of fat and sugar
> - Eat regular meals as a family
> - Eat breakfast
> - Watch the portion sizes and how often food is eaten

can be achieved with the help of a dietitian, but this is only helpful if it is sustainable. Self-monitoring and rewards for reaching goals are useful. Adoption of healthy eating by the whole family, especially if other members are overweight, is effective (Box 16.1). Cooperation of the child and the whole family is essential (Figures 16.3 and 16.4).

Increasing exercise

A practical objective is to increase physical activity by at least 60 minutes each day although not necessarily at one time. Sedentary behaviour such as watching television, using a computer, or playing video games should be confined to 1 hour per day. The choice of physical activity should be agreed with the child and may involve informal exercise such as walking to school, cycling, or climbing stairs instead of using a lift. Regular structured activity may include sports at school, football, swimming, or dancing. Activity of the whole family should be increased by walking to the local shops or park together.

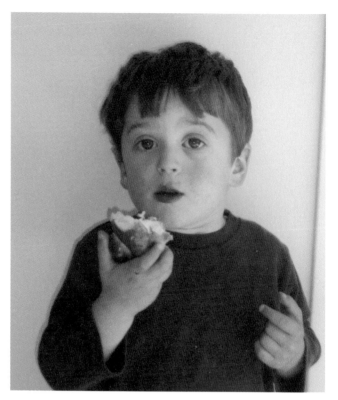

Figure 16.3 Bread is healthy.

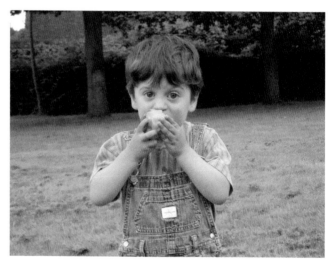

Figure 16.4 Fruit is healthy.

Support

Obese children are often the victims of teasing or bullying by peers and psychological disturbance is common. Psychological support is needed during and after attempts to lose weight.

Further reading

National Institute for Clinical Excellence (NICE). *Obesity*. NICE Guideline CG 43, 2006. www.nice.org.uk

Valman B. *When Your Child is Ill: a Home Guide for Parents*, 3rd edn. Dorling Kindersley, London, 2008.

CHAPTER 17

Common Rashes

Bernard Valman

Northwick Park Hospital and Imperial College London, UK

OVERVIEW

- Rashes usually occur as part of one of the common infectious diseases of childhood, but these must be distinguished from dermatological causes.
- The characteristics of the lesions, distribution, changes with time, and accompanying features help to make the diagnosis. An accurate description of the rash limits the number of diagnoses that need to be considered.
- A previous attack of an infectious disease makes a further attack unlikely, but a high incidence of wrong diagnoses of some rashes detracts from the value of this history.

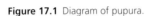

Figure 17.1 Diagram of pupura.

Purpura

Purpuric lesions are caused by haemorrhages in the skin and do not disappear on pressure (Figures 17.1 and 17.2). Children with purpura usually need to be admitted to hospital immediately as they may have meningococcal septicaemia (Figure 17.2), leukaemia, or idiopathic thrombocytopenic purpura. Henoch–Schönlein purpura is more common than these conditions, however, and is distributed over the extensor surfaces of the limbs as well as the buttocks, and some of the purpuric lesions are raised (Figures 17.3 and 17.4). If the rash has all the features characteristic of Henoch–Schönlein purpura then admission to hospital is not needed.

Macules and papules

Macules are discrete lesions that change the colour of the skin, although they fade on pressure (Figures 17.5 and 17.6). They may be of any size or shape and may be pink or red.

Discrete, pink, minute macules occur in rubella, when they are accompanied by suboccipital lymphadenopathy. In both

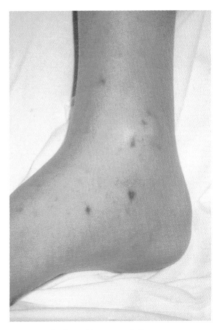

Figure 17.2 Pupuric rash of meningococcal disease.

roseola and rubella suboccipital lymphadenopathy is pronounced, but in roseola the appearance of the rash coincides with the disappearance of all other symptoms. The child with rubella may have slight fever. In contrast, infants with roseola have high fever and irritability for 3 or 4 days before the macular rash appears (see p. 65). Despite the high fever the child may play normally.

Papules are solid palpable projections above the surface of the skin (Figures 17.7 and 17.8). Insect bites are one cause of these lesions, which are called papular urticaria.

ABC of One to Seven, 5th edition. Edited by B. Valman. © 2010 Blackwell Publishing, ISBN: 978-1-4051-8105-1.

Figure 17.3 Diagram of Henoch–Schönlein purpura.

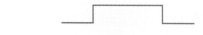

Figure 17.7 Diagram of papule.

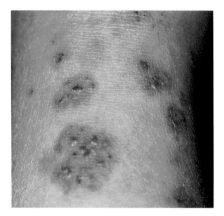

Figure 17.4 Henoch–Schönlein purpura.

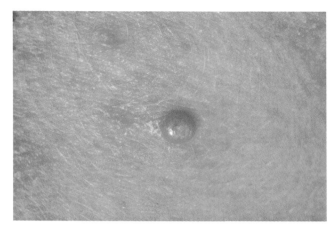

Figure 17.8 Papule.

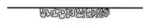

Figure 17.5 Diagram of macule.

Maculopapular rash

A maculopapular rash is a mixture of the two types of lesion described above, which tend to be confluent (Figure 17.9). A maculopapular rash is the typical rash of measles (Figure 17.10), when it is always accompanied by cough and sometimes by nasal discharge. The most common problem is to distinguish measles from a drug rash, which may itch. Koplik spots have usually disappeared by this stage, but if they persist they may be helpful. The drug may have been given for an upper respiratory tract infection and the clinical picture may mimic measles.

A maculopapular rash occurs in glandular fever, especially in patients who have received ampicillin or one of its derivatives. Patients who have been receiving ampicillin may develop a drug rash during their first course of treatment. The rash usually occurs about day 10 after starting the drug. Usually, a second exposure after an interval is needed for a drug rash to occur.

Vesicles

Vesicles are blisters caused by fluid raising the horny layer of the epidermis (Figure 17.11). In chickenpox the lesions pass through the stages of macule, papule, and vesicle within 2 days and crops of rash occur (Figure 17.12). A fairly clear vesicle on the skin is the diagnostic lesion. Vesicles change to pustules and later to scales or ulcers.

In herpes zoster vesicles occur in the distribution of a sensory nerve. Itching may occur before the rash appears.

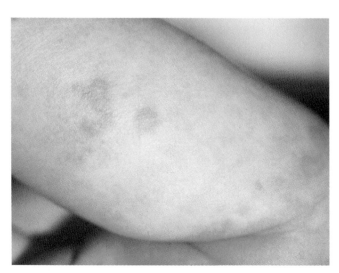

Figure 17.6 Macular rash of meningococcal disease.

An infant's first contact with herpes simplex virus may cause vesicles and severe ulcers in the mouth or on the vulva or conjunctiva.

Summer outbreaks of hand, foot, and mouth disease are recognized by the pearly white vesicles at these sites, which are caused by a Coxsackie virus.

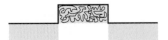

Figure 17.9 Diagram of maculopapular rash.

Figure 17.10 Maculopapular rash (measles).

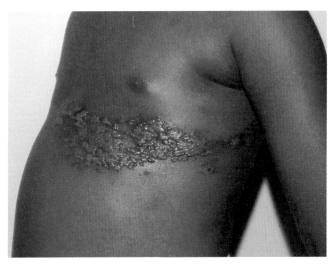

Figure 17.11 Vesicles (herpes zoster).

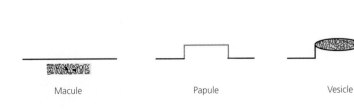

Macule Papule Vesicle Crusting Ulcer

Figure 17.12 Progression of rash in chickenpox.

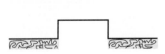

Figure 17.13 Diagram of wheal.

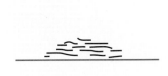

Figure 17.14 Diagram of desquamation.

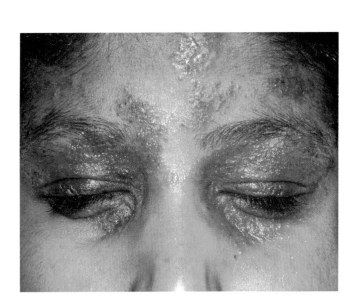

Figure 17.15 Desquamation.

Wheals

Wheals are raised lesions with a pale centre surrounded by a red area (Figure 17.13). The rash is accompanied by itching, and the cause is usually not discovered. The rash may be difficult to diagnose in the resolving phase.

Desquamation

Desquamation is a loss of epidermal cells which produces a 'scaly' eruption (Figure 17.14). Desquamation is found in atopic eczema and affects the flexures, face, and neck but may be more widespread (Figure 17.15). Psoriasis produces round, scaly lesions 0.5–1.0 cm in diameter on the face, trunk, and limbs.

Further reading

Harper J, Oranje A, Prose N. *Textbook of Paediatric Dermatology*, 2nd edn. Blackwell Publishing, Oxford, 2005.

CHAPTER 18

Infectious Diseases

Bernard Valman

Northwick Park Hospital and Imperial College London, UK

OVERVIEW

- The prevalence of the majority of the infectious diseases of childhood have been considerably reduced or eliminated by immunization.
- The reduction in immunization rates as a result of ill-informed adverse publicity may cause resurgence of these diseases.
- Frequent travel to parts of the world with low prevalence of immunization may cause children to present with diseases that are rarely seen in this country.
- When a receptionist receives a request for a child with a new rash to be seen, arrangements should be made for the family to be directed to a special room on arrival rather than wait in the main waiting area.

Measles

After an incubation period of 8–14 days there is a prodromal illness with cough, fever, and nasal discharge (Figure 18.1). The presence of a cough is essential for the diagnosis. During the prodromal period there are minute white spots on a red background on the buccal mucosa opposite the molar teeth (Koplik spots). After about 4 days a maculopapular rash appears on the face and behind the ears and spreads downwards to cover the whole body while older lesions become more blotchy (Figure 18.2). As the rash appears the Koplik spots fade. The rash begins to fade after 3–4 days and is accompanied by a fall in temperature and a reduction in malaise. Some children become irritable. Measles is not contagious after the fifth day of the rash (Table 18.1), but exposure has usually occurred before the diagnosis is obvious. Attempts to isolate siblings from each other are useless.

Acute otitis media is the most common complication of measles; signs usually appear about 3 days after the onset of the rash. Antibiotics should be given if these signs appear but there is no place for prophylactic antibiotics against otitis media. The onset of bronchopneumonia may be difficult to detect as a severe cough is part of the measles. A raised respiratory rate at rest or added sounds are confirmatory signs. The serious complication of encephalitis

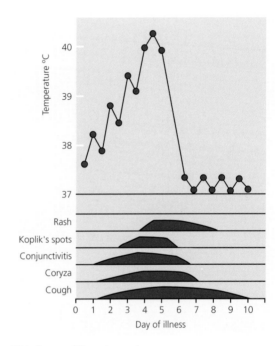

Figure 18.1 Course of illness in measles.

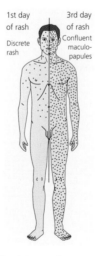

Figure 18.2 Distribution of rash in measles.

Table 18.1 Advice for contacts and exclusion from school or nursery.

Infection	Advice for contacts (from haematologist)	Exclusion from school or nursery
Chickenpox	Compromised immunity e.g. leukaemia	Until lesions crust (5–7 days)
Measles	Chronic lung or heart disease (inform paediatrician)	5 days after onset of rash
Rubella	Pregnancy (inform obstetrician)	7 days after onset of rash
Fifth disease	Haemolytic anaemia Pregnancy (inform obstetrician)	Nil
Scarlet fever	Nil	Until rash has resolved
Roseola	Nil	Nil

a few hours. During the illness the child seems to be less ill than might be expected from the height of the fever, but pronounced irritability may suggest the possibility of meningitis. The suboccipital, cervical, and postauricular lymph nodes are often enlarged and there is often neutropenia. Some children have mild diarrhoea, cough, or pain in the ear. A child with a suppressed immune system may develop hepatitis or pneumonia. Most children have had the illness, with or without the rash, by the time they are 2 years old. Roseola is caused by human herpesvirus 6 or 7.

Chickenpox

After an incubation period of 14–17 days the rash appears on the trunk and face (Figure 18.4). The spots appear in crops passing from macule to papule, vesicle, and pustule within 2 days. Lesions in the mouth produce painful, shallow ulcers and if they are in the trachea and bronchi may produce a severe cough (Figure 18.5).

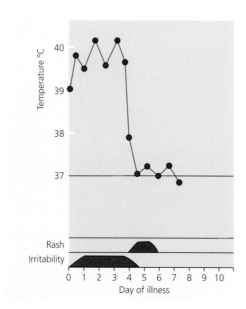

Figure 18.3 Roseola.

occurs in about 1 in 1000 affected children and causes drowsiness, vomiting, headache, and convulsions about 7 days after the onset of measles. In developing countries measles has a high morbidity and mortality, and diarrhoea is a common feature, particularly in severely malnourished children.

A drug reaction in the presence of a viral infection is difficult to distinguish from measles rash. Features suggesting a drug reaction are lack of cough, an irritating rash, or an atypical distribution of spots.

Roseola

Following an incubation period of 5–15 days, there is high fever which is a notorious feature of roseola infantum (Figure 18.3). There may be a convulsion at the onset. The temperature usually reaches 39–40°C and remains at this level for 3–4 days. The temperature falls and the child becomes well as discrete, minute, pink macules appear on the trunk; these may spread to the limbs within

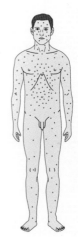

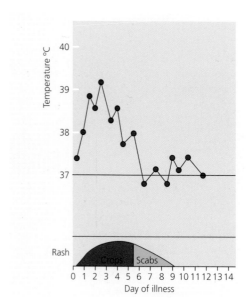

Figure 18.4 Distribution of rash in chickenpox.

Figure 18.5 Course of illness in chickenpox.

Severe irritation of the skin may occur and may be alleviated by calamine lotion and oral promethazine. The lesions normally pass through a pustular stage, and as this is not bacterial in origin, local or oral antibiotics are rarely required. Encephalitis is rare but often produces cerebellar signs with ataxia. This occurs 3–8 days after the onset of the rash, and most patients recover completely.

Secondarily infected lesions and scabs removed by scratching may be followed by scarring. Red areas round some lesions indicate secondary infection usually with group A streptococci and an antibiotic is indicated. A child with chickenpox may transmit the disease to other susceptible children from 1 day before the onset of the rash until all the vesicles have crusted. The dry scabs do not contain active virus. Complete crusting of the lesions occurs 5–10 days after onset. Chickenpox may be contracted from a patient with herpes zoster.

If a child with compromised immunity – for example, one being treated for acute leukaemia – is in contact with a child with chickenpox and has not previously contracted that disease, advice should be sought on whether zoster immunoglobulin should be given for prophylaxis. If chickenpox occurs in an immunocompromised child then urgent admission to hospital for intravenous aciclovir is indicated. A child with atopic eczema and chickenpox may be given oral aciclovir.

Scarlet fever

Scarlet fever is less virulent than it was in the mid-1900s. Sequelae such as rheumatic fever and acute glomerulonephritis are very rare. It is caused by an erythrogenic strain of group A haemolytic streptococci. After an incubation period of 2–4 days fever, headache, and tonsillitis appear (Figure 18.6). Pinpoint macules which blanch on pressure occur on the trunk and neck with increased density in the neck, axillae, and groins (Figure 18.7). A thick, white coating on the tongue peels on the third day, leaving a 'strawberry' appearance. The rash lasts about 6 days and is followed by peeling. A 10-day course of oral penicillin eradicates the organism and may prevent other children from being infected.

Fifth disease (erythema infectiosum)

Fifth disease is caused by parvovirus B19 and usually occurs in small outbreaks in children over the age of 2 years in the spring. Mild systemic symptoms are accompanied by an intensely red appearance of the face, with circumoral pallor, which is called 'slapped cheek' syndrome. A symmetrical maculopapular lace-like rash is noted on the arms, moving downwards to involve the trunk, buttocks, and thighs (Figure 18.8). The rash can recur and fluctuate in intensity with environmental changes, such as temperature and exposure to sunlight, for weeks or months. Arthralgia and arteritis occur infrequently in children but more commonly in young women.

In patients with haemolytic anaemia – for example, sickle cell disease – the virus may cause an aplastic crisis lasting 7–10 days, but with no rash.

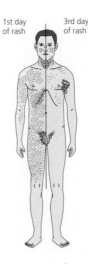

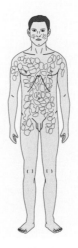

Figure 18.7 Distribution of rash in scarlet fever.

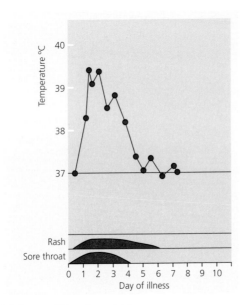

Figure 18.6 Course of illness in scarlet fever.

Figure 18.8 Distribution of rash in fifth disease.

Parvovirus infection during early pregnancy causes fetal death in less than 10% of cases, and no congenital anomalies have been reported.

The incubation period is usually 4–14 days, and children are unlikely to be infectious after the onset of the rash.

Rubella

Rubella or German measles is usually a mild illness and the rash may not be noticed. The incidence of rubella infections without rash may be 25%. When a rash does occur it appears as a pink, minute, discrete, macular rash on the face and trunk after an incubation period of 14–21 days (Figure 18.9). The suboccipital lymph nodes are enlarged and there may be generalized lymphadenopathy (Figure 18.10). Thrombocytopenia, encephalitis, and arthritis are rare complications of rubella. The period of infectivity probably extends from the latter part of the incubation period to the end of the first week of the rash.

If rubella occurs during the first 5 months of pregnancy the fetus may die or develop congenital heart disease, mental retardation, deafness, or cataracts. If any rash occurs during pregnancy a specimen of blood should be taken immediately and again 10 days later for measuring rubella antibody titres to determine whether a recent infection with rubella has occurred.

Whooping cough

Whooping cough is discussed on p. 11.

Infectious mononucleosis

This disease can occur at any age but is most common in adolescents and young adults. It is caused by the Epstein–Barr virus. After an incubation period of 30–50 days there is fever which may last from a few days to several weeks. There is often a sore throat which may be severe. Localized or generalized lymphadenopathy may be accompanied by a maculopapular rash affecting the face and trunk. Hepatitis is the most common complication, but there may be central nervous system involvement, myocarditis, or orchitis in severe cases. A full blood count and blood screening test confirms the diagnosis.

Most children return to school after 2 weeks but a few may need to return only part time for a few more weeks. More prolonged fatigue may occur in a small proportion of children when the possibility of chronic fatigue syndrome should be considered (see p. 106).

Mumps

Following an incubation period of 14–21 days there is fever and swelling of one or both parotid glands, which may be painful. The swelling lasts 4–8 days. Occasionally, adolescent boys develop orchitis a week after the parotid swelling started, but it is usually unilateral and rarely causes infertility. Torsion of the testis should be excluded (see p. 30). Rarely, encephalitis, meningitis, or pancreatitis may occur, either before or after the swelling of the parotid glands. Rarely, mumps is followed by permanent hearing loss.

Typhoid fever

Typhoid fever is caused by *Salmonella typhi* which is acquired from food or water contaminated with infected stools. After an incubation period of 7–14 days the following may appear:
- Fever that rises gradually to 39–40°C and stays at this level without daily fluctuations for up to 4 weeks;
- Headache;
- Lack of energy;
- Abdominal pain;
- Constipation or diarrhoea;
- Raised pink lesions on the abdomen and chest which appear in the second week of the illness and last about a day;
- Intestinal bleeding or perforation in the second or third week if no treatment has been given.

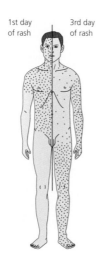

Figure 18.9 Distribution of rash in rubella.

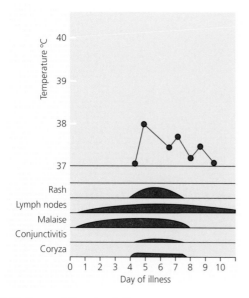

Figure 18.10 Course of illness in rubella.

Following admission to an isolation bed in hospital, the diagnosis is confirmed by culture of blood, stool, and urine. An antibiotic is given as soon as the cultures have been taken, but there may be an interval of several days before the symptoms resolve. Immunization is available before travel to countries where the disease is common.

HIV and AIDS

Most children with HIV (human immunodeficiency virus) are infected from their mothers before birth. Initially, the infection produces few symptoms, but it progressively damages the immune system causing AIDS (acquired immune deficiency syndrome). Most infants infected in the perinatal period have symptoms before the age of 2 years but the first symptoms may appear as late as 12 years.

There are a wide range of symptoms including:

- Failure to thrive;
- Recurrent diarrhoea;
- Enlarged lymph nodes;
- Recurrent *Candida* infections;
- Recurrent and severe pneumonia;
- Developmental delay.

The diagnosis should be considered if the mother has a positive antenatal screening test or the infant has one or more of the features above. Counselling is arranged for both parents and, if they agree, a blood test is performed on the infant. Although the mother's HIV antibodies may remain in the infant's blood for a year or more, another test can confirm or exclude the infection in the first few months of life.

A combination of drugs is given against the virus to slow development of the disease, but resistance of the virus to drugs and the toxicity of the drugs limit effective treatment. Antibacterial drugs such as co-trimoxazole may be used to prevent or control opportunistic infection such as pneumonia.

If treatment is given during pregnancy and breastfeeding is avoided, the risk of transmitting the infection is less than 1%.

Further reading

Isaacs D. *Evidence Based Paediatric Infectious Diseases.* Blackwell Publishing, Oxford, 2007.

CHAPTER 19

Paediatric Dermatology

Saleem Goolamali

Clementine Churchill Hospital, Harrow, UK

Atopic dermatitis (eczema)

The word eczema is derived from the Greek word elements *ec* (out and over), *ze* (boiling) and *ma* (the result of) which relate to the tiny vesicles that form in the acute stage of the condition. 'Atopy' from the Greek *a, top* and *y* 'without a place' so called because when the word was employed there was no classification available and hence 'no place' for the genuine association of this form of dermatitis with 'hayfever' (now allergic rhinitis) and asthma (reactive airways disease). In practice, the words eczema and dermatitis, which have different connotations for the etymologist, are used interchangeably by clinicians.

In the UK atopic dermatitis develops in some 15–20% of school-age children usually before the age of 5 years. The dermatitis occurs alone in approximately 54% of patients, dermatitis with asthma in 12%, dermatitis with allergic rhinitis in 12%, and the triad of dermatitis, allergic rhinitis, and asthma in 22%.

Atopic dermatitis is characterized by pruritus and erythematous vesicular lesions with a distinct predilection for the face and the skin creases – folds of elbows, behind the knees, and the neck (Figure 19.1). In around 60% of children a remission occurs in adolescence but recurrence in adulthood is not infrequent. Atopic children have a lower threshold to pruritic stimuli and some children are worse during cold weather. Ultraviolet light, more recently narrow band UVB, used under specialist supervision is a potent ancillary treatment for severe cases. Many parents report an improvement in their child's dermatitis in the sun but exposure to sunlight needs to be measured as sunburn will exacerbate dermatitis and heat from any source can trigger itch. Woollen clothing also irritates atopic skin.

Controversy continues to exist in atopic dermatitis regarding the role of allergens in ingested foods and airborne allergens such as house dust, moulds, and dander, and mites in the fur of family pets such as dogs and cats. It is commonly accepted that the diagnosis of food-induced dermatitis requires a positive and persisting response after challenge. Measurements of total serum immunoglobulin E (IgE) and tests for antibodies to allergens (RAST) can be distinctly unhelpful. Some 15% of apparently normal individuals have elevated IgE levels while 20% of patients with typical atopic dermatitis have normal levels of IgE and negative RAST tests. Unsupported overzealous food restriction may result in malnutrition.

In infants and young children the itch and discomfort, and the loss of sleep it causes, allied with the social stigma of atopic dermatitis allow little room for experimentation with unpleasant medications of uncertain effect. The mode of action of traditional Chinese herbal medicine is unclear although some eczema patients have responded temporarily. It is important to emphasize that even 'natural' herbs can occasionally have serious side effects and liver and renal damage have been recorded.

The initial consultation therefore needs to be unhurried and optimistic. The family expects a cure or at the very least tests to 'find the allergy'. Time taken to explain the nature of atopic dermatitis and the rationale for the choice of treatment helps to form a team approach. Parents should be advised to allow their children to receive the full immunization programme.

Topical steroids used correctly remain the only consistently effective, predominantly safe therapy for atopic dermatitis. Many parents are averse to the use of topical steroids having learnt of side effects from a variety of well-wishers and nowadays the Internet. The fact that topical steroids have different levels of potency – mild, moderately potent, potent, and very potent – is important to discuss with the added reassurance that as far as possible preparations in the mild category are employed for children. An open and honest approach to the limitations of treatment should form part of the therapy and any misconceptions regarding the use of topical steroids clarified. Failure to do so inevitably results in non-compliance and an unhappy and disillusioned family.

1% Hydrocortisone, a mild topical steroid, is safe in children but overuse of potent or very potent topical steroids can cause telangiectasia and striae especially over thin-skin areas. Children should be prescribed sufficient cream or ointment to treat the areas affected. If only a small amount is given it can reinforce the impression that the medication is 'strong' and possibly harmful.

Failure of dermatitis to respond when it has previously been well controlled should raise the possibility of a contact allergy or secondary bacterial or viral infection. *Staphylococcus aureus* is the infecting organism in the vast majority and is nearly always

ABC of One to Seven, 5th edition. Edited by B. Valman. © 2010 Blackwell Publishing, ISBN: 978-1-4051-8105-1.

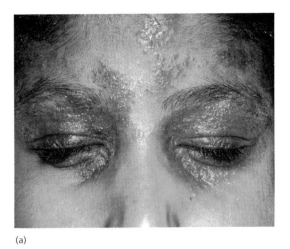

(a)

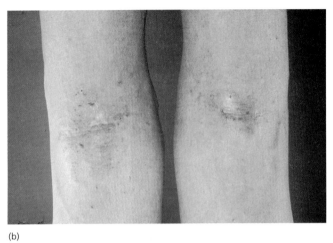

(b)

Figure 19.1 (a) Acute infected atopic eczema. (b) Atopic eczema commonly affects knee flexures.

penicillin resistant. In the absence of allergy oral erythromycin is a reasonable first choice of antibiotic. Nocturnal itching can be reduced with an antihistamine such as alimemazine (trimeprazine) or hydroxyzine hydrochloride. One of the mainstays of long-term management is the frequent use of bland emollients. Creams and ointments are better in this respect than lotions. Patients should be advised to avoid medicated soap but a mild moisturising soap or non-soap cleanser may be used. Additionally lubricants which help to moisten and soften the skin are best applied immediately after bathing while the skin is still moist.

Topical calcineurin inhibitors – tacrolimus and pimecrolimus – are recommended as options for atopic eczema not controlled by optimal treatment with topical corticosteroid therapy or if there is a risk of important corticosteroid-related side effects, in particular skin atrophy. These treatments at present are best considered second line therapy and then prescribed by those experienced in treating atopic eczema.

Eczema herpeticum (Kaposi's varicelliform eruption)

Herpes simplex virus (HSV) may complicate active or resolving atopic eczema. The usual mode of acquisition is through direct exposure of abraded skin to the lesions of an individual with active primary or recurrent HSV infection. Kaposi's varicelliform eruption is a rapidly forming vesicular eruption that occurs mainly on abnormal skin but can become generalized (Figure 19.2). It is an indication for urgent referral to hospital. Fever and lymphadenopathy are usually present and there may be ocular and neurological complications. Patients should be isolated and receive antibiotics to prevent secondary bacterial infection. In addition, aciclovir is prescribed for topical use preferably within 48 hours of the eruption. Aciclovir, famciclovir, and valaciclovir are safe and effective oral antiviral agents. Aciclovir, available also as an intravenous infusion, may be indicated if the infection is severe or if there are neurological complications. Steroids, both topical and systemic, should be avoided although pre-existing systemic steroid treatment should not be stopped suddenly.

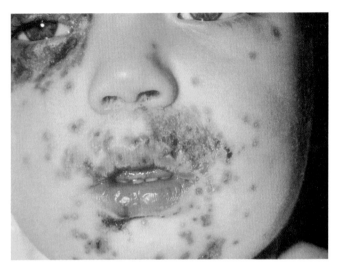

Figure 19.2 Eczema herpeticum.

Impetigo

Impetigo contagiosa is an infectious superficial infection usually caused, in temperate climates, by staphylococci or by mixed invasion by streptococci and staphylococci. In infants it can cause severe illness but in adults it is usually trivial. It often develops as a complication of a skin condition, especially eczema, but also commonly accompanies pediculosis or scabies. In the common variety superficial, thin-roofed lakes of pus form on the face, hands, or knees and evolve rapidly into raw, oozing areas which dry, leaving golden crusts (Figure 19.3). In the bullous variety large, thick-walled blisters appear. The contents are initially clear but later purulent. The crusts should be removed gently by soaking with saline solution. The raw areas are then treated with a thin smear of mupirocin (Bactroban) three times daily for 7 days and an oral antibiotic is given. The child should stay at home until the eruption has cleared. In recurrent impetigo look for staphylococci in the nose in otherwise asymptomatic individuals. If present, intranasal mupirocin is indicated.

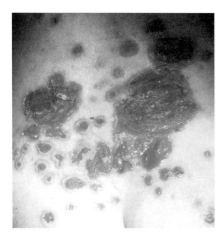

Figure 19.3 Impetigo.

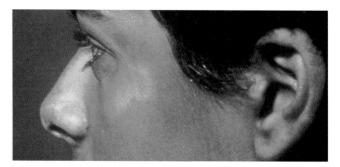

Figure 19.5 Pityriasis alba.

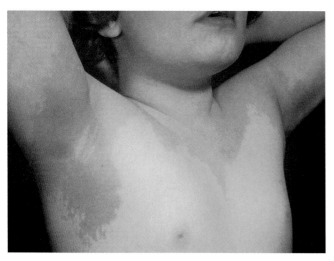

Figure 19.4 Seborrhoeic dermatitis.

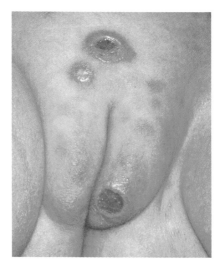

Figure 19.6 Napkin dermatitis.

Seborrhoeic dermatitis

Seborrhoeic dermatitis is so called because it occurs in sites of increased sebaceous activity: the face, neck, chest, and back. However, seborrhoea, or an abnormality of the sebaceous glands, is not considered a feature of the condition. It occurs commonly in the first 3 months of life as an erythematous, scaly eruption on the scalp and face, but any of the body folds may be affected, including the neck, axillae, and groin (Figure 19.4). There is no itching but secondary infection is common, particularly with *Candida*. In some children atopic dermatitis may follow seborrhoeic dermatitis, but the latter is not thought to be caused by atopy. Low potency topical steroids combined with an anti-*Candida* preparation are helpful in the treatment of seborrhoeic dermatitis. For the scalp an anti-seborrhoeic shampoo is useful.

Pityriasis alba

Pityriasis alba is a form of dermatitis that occurs predominantly in children as rounded or oval, hypopigmented, mildly scaly patches, usually on the face but occasionally on the upper arms and back (Figure 19.5). It may be associated with atopic eczema or may occur alone. The patches are often multiple, and initial erythema is followed by hypopigmentation, which prompts the parents to seek advice. The eruption is self-limiting but may last 2–3 years. Pityriasis alba must be differentiated from vitiligo. The scaling may be reduced by a bland cream and any inflammation treated with a weak topical steroid, such as hydrocortisone.

Napkin dermatitis (contact irritant type)

Neonatal skin is thinner than adult skin, has less eccrine and sebaceous gland secretions, but is more susceptible to external irritants and bacterial infection, and these can combine with other factors to produce 'contact' dermatitis.

Prolonged contact with urine or faeces, maceration of skin induced by wet napkins and waterproof pants, and secondary infection with *Candida albicans* lead to an irritant dermatitis. Urea-splitting bacteria which release ammonia are encouraged by the warm, wet environment produced by impervious clothing. The dermatitis appears as a confluent erythema at sites closest to the napkin, usually with sparing of the folds, and readily becomes secondarily infected, producing pustules and erosions (Figure 19.6). In boys inflammation of the urethral

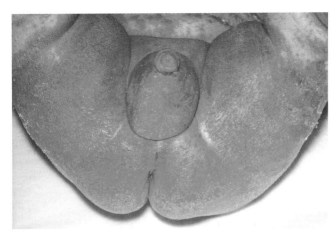

Figure 19.7 Napkin dermatitis.

meatus often occurs and may cause dysuria and urinary retention (Figure 19.7).

Napkin dermatitis is managed by keeping the area clean and dry and avoiding occlusive dressings. Plastic or rubber pants should not be used except for important occasions. Disposable napkins are preferable to those that require plastic overpants, although some disposable napkins also have an outer plastic lining. Towelling napkins are best if thoroughly washed, rinsed, and sterilized. A mild detergent is advisable and the rinse cycle of the washing machine needs to be completed twice. Napkins must be changed often. Regular compresses of saline solution (one level teaspoon of salt in a pint of water) can be applied if the dermatitis is acute and exudative, or alternatively the affected area can be exposed for 2–3 days. In the past ointments have been avoided for acute weeping dermatoses but they are as effective as creams when used in similar concentrations. A 1% hydrocortisone preparation is used three or four times daily for a week, but a more potent steroid such as triamcinolone may be necessary for severe dermatitis. Strong fluorinated steroids should be used only under specialist supervision. Secondary bacterial infection is treated with both topical and oral antibiotics. Similarly, monilial infection is treated by topical nystatin, and oral nystatin is also given to clear the intestinal reservoir of yeast. When the skin has recovered a barrier preparation such as zinc ointment BP is applied with each nappy change to prevent recurrence. Preparations that contain arachis (peanut) oil should be avoided in case the child has a peanut allergy.

'Lick' eczema

The site of a contact irritant dermatitis varies according to the cause. A reaction to a perfumed spray or a bubble bath may cause a widespread eruption, although the rash is often most prominent on the cheeks, neck, external surfaces of the limbs, and the buttocks. Lip licking or thumb sucking often causes a reaction due to saliva (Figure 19.8). The child and parents do not recognize the cause but notice a spreading, irritating, perioral

eruption with fissuring of the skin. Explanation of the aetiology together with a mild topical steroid for a few days and then liberal applications of petroleum jelly especially before sleep help to clear the eruption.

Warts

Human warts are caused by the human papillomavirus, a member of the papovavirus group to which children aged 6–12 years are particularly prone. Sixty five per cent resolve within 2 years of their onset. Warts may occur anywhere on the body and four types are recognised: common, plane (Figure 19.9), plantar, and genital warts. Genital warts can be sexually transmitted but not necessarily so. Innocent transmission of common warts to the genital area may occur via infected carers during activities such as bathing the child or changing napkins. Most warts occur on the hands and feet and children who are immunosuppressed and those with atopic dermatitis are particularly susceptible to warts and molluscum contagiosum. Warts may develop at sites of trauma (Koebner phenomenon). The verruca will often show multiple, thrombosed, capillary loops which resemble black dots (Figure 19.10).

Warts are destroyed by physical or chemical methods. The adage that the best way to manage warts is to let them manage themselves still seems appropriate. When treatment is necessary

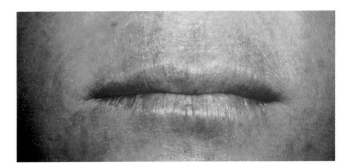

Figure 19.8 Lick eczema.

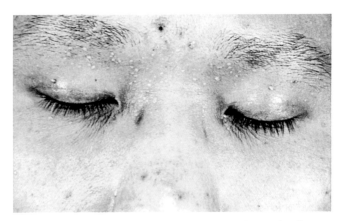

Figure 19.9 Multiple plane warts in older children may be mistaken for acne vulgaris.

simple procedures such as covering the lesion with a waterproof, adhesive bandage changed daily should be tried initially. The next measure is to pare the surface of the wart with an emery board or pumice stone, and apply a keratolytic preparation such as salicylic acid daily for up to 12 weeks. A little petroleum jelly smeared on the normal skin around the wart will protect it from any irritant effect. If these methods fail the wart may be frozen with liquid nitrogen as this avoids the need for local anaesthetic and does not produce the painful scar that often results from diathermy, cautery, or excision.

Molluscum contagiosum

Molluscum contagiosum is caused by a virus of the family Poxviridae. The virus is passed directly by skin contact but transmission via fomites on bath sponges and bath towels has been implicated as a source of infection. As the name implies, the lesions can spread rapidly. Multiple lesions are common in young children between the age of 2 and 5 years and tend to occur frequently on the trunk and less commonly on the extremities and face. The typical lesion is a dome-shaped, flesh-coloured, umbilicated papule which releases a cheesy, white material when pierced and expressed (Figure 19.11).

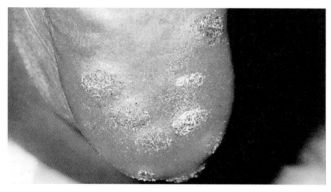

Figure 19.10 Plantar verucae.

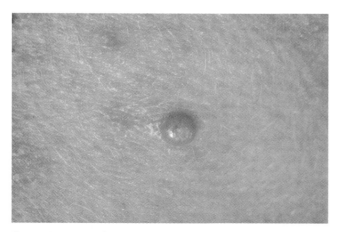

Figure 19.11 Dome-shaped umbilicated papule of molluscum.

Molluscum contagiosum can resolve spontaneously but spread of lesions, particularly to the face, demands treatment. The lesions may be readily destroyed by piercing with a sharp orange stick and, depending on the site of infection, dipped in an anti-wart paint. Other equally effective measures include gentle cryotherapy and curettage. With multiple lesions topical tretinoin (Retin-A) has been found to be successful in some patients. In order to prevent autoinoculation simultaneous treatment of all molluscum lesions present is prudent.

Pediculosis capitis

The agent of head louse infestation *Pediculus humanus capitis* most commonly infects the scalp of children 3–11 years of age. The egg-filled capsules, nits (Figure 19.12a), and lice are attached to the hair of the head and eyelashes (Figure 19.12b) and there may be secondary impetigo of the scalp. The adult female louse lays some 5–10 eggs a day during her lifespan of 30 days. Generally the eggs are laid within 1 cm of the scalp surface.

Traditionally, it is recommended that nits and lice are removed either manually or with a fine-toothed comb. The removal of all nits from a child's scalp can take several hours. Permethrin and phenothrin are pyrethroids, both of which are effective treatments but lice have developed resistance in some districts. Treatment should preferably be repeated after 7 days to clear any lice emerging from any eggs that might have survived the first application. Some health districts operate a rotating policy for head lice treatment. In view of increasing resistance, however, any doubt about the efficacy of a product should lead to the use of another one. Malathion is also recommended for head lice. It is important in all cases to read the manufacturer's instructions especially when prescribing for children. The vast majority of head louse infections are acquired by direct head-to-head contact but children should be persuaded to avoid sharing each others' brushes or combs as head lice may occasionally be spread by sharing infested grooming items. Eyelash infestation can be treated with petrolatum applied to the eyelid margin twice daily for 8 days which asphyxiates the parasites.

Scabies

Scabies is caused by the ubiquitous mite *Sarcoptes scabiei*, a six-legged arthropod (Figure 19.13a) which causes the typical eruption of pruritic papules, vesicles, and burrows (Figure 19.13b). The papules result from invasion of the larval stages of the parasite, the vesicles from host sensitisation, and the burrow marks the site of the adult female mite where it has dug into the horny layer of the epidermis. In adults and older children the eruption tends to favour the finger webs, flexor aspects of the wrists, axillae, and the genitalia. In infants and young children the distribution may include the palms and soles, the head, face, and neck, and burrows may be absent (Figure 19.13c). Furthermore, bullae, which are uncommon in the adult, may occur in children.

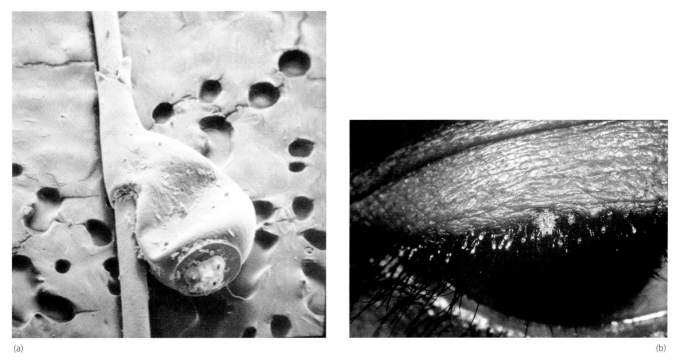

(a)

(b)

Figure 19.12 (a) Head louse egg attached to hair shaft. (b) Lice infestation of eyelashes.

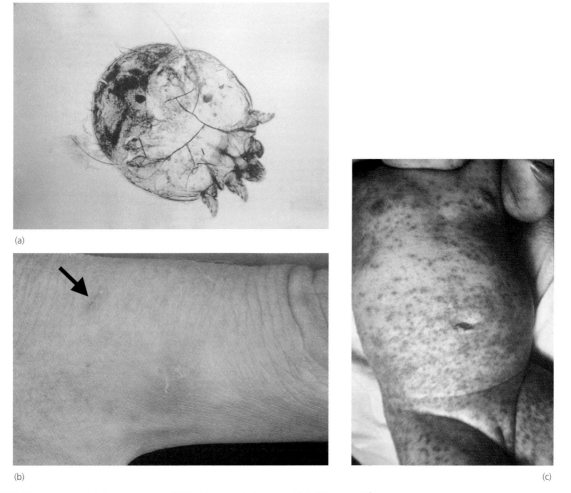

(a)

(b)

(c)

Figure 19.13 (a) Sarcoptes scabiei, the scabies mite. (b) Scabies – classic burrows. (c) Scabies in an infant.

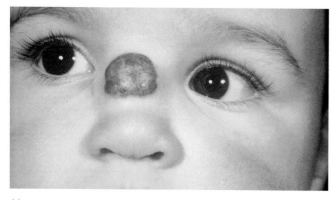

(a)

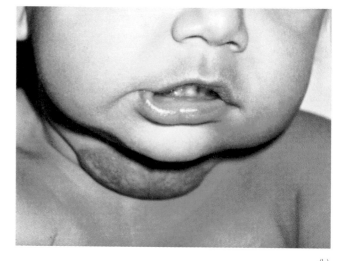

(b)

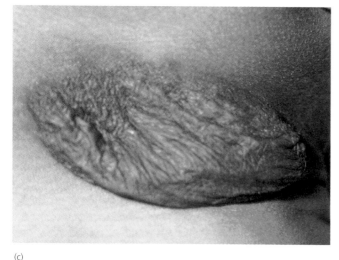

(c)

Figure 19.14 (a) Strawberry haemangioma. (b) Haemangioma under chin. (c) Redundant skin associated with resolving haemangioma.

Permethrin has largely replaced lindane for the treatment of scabies. It is highly effective and appears also to be much safer. The preparation is applied over the whole body and washed off after 8 hours. In children the cream may also be applied to the face, neck, scalp, and ears. If the hands are washed with soap and water within 8 hours of application the cream should be reapplied. All people occupying the same accommodation and others in close contact should be treated even if they do not show overt evidence of scabies. At the end of treatment, because mites can survive for as long as 48 hours off the host, intimate articles of clothing (underwear, pyjamas, sheets, and pillowcases) should be laundered and ironed. Even after adequate treatment pruritus may persist but this usually responds to 10% crotamiton cream used for a week or two. If this appears unsuccessful reinfection or an alternative cause should be considered.

Vascular anomalies

Modern classification of vascular anomalies divides them into vascular tumours and vascular malformations. Congenital and infantile haemangiomas are classified as vascular tumours whereas a port-wine stain (capillary haemangioma, naevus flammeus) is now described as a vascular (capillary) malformation.

Vascular tumours – haemangiomas – are the most common tumours in children, occurring in some 10%. They are more common in girls and are normally seen on the head and neck. Cavernous haemangiomas (strawberry) are not present at birth but start to become apparent within the first month of life (Figure 19.14a). The angioma is usually solitary but often grows rapidly for several months to achieve maximal size after about a year. It is situated commonly in the upper dermis but large lesions may extend into subcutaneous tissue. They are initially dark red, tense, and shiny but soon start to involute. This is heralded by a diminution of redness and a white–grey fibrosis which develops within the lesion (Figure 19.14b,c). A rule of thumb is that 50% resolve by the age of 5 years, 70% by the age of 7 years, and 90% by 9 years. The superficial variety clears completely whereas deeper lesions may show only partial resolution and could require corrective surgery. Pulse dye laser therapy can be helpful with rapidly growing superficial haemangiomas that ulcerate. Haemangiomas that expand to cover the nose or the eye are of concern as they can interfere with vision, feeding, and breathing. This may then require treatment with prednisolone 2–3 mg/kg/day over a 3–4 week period.

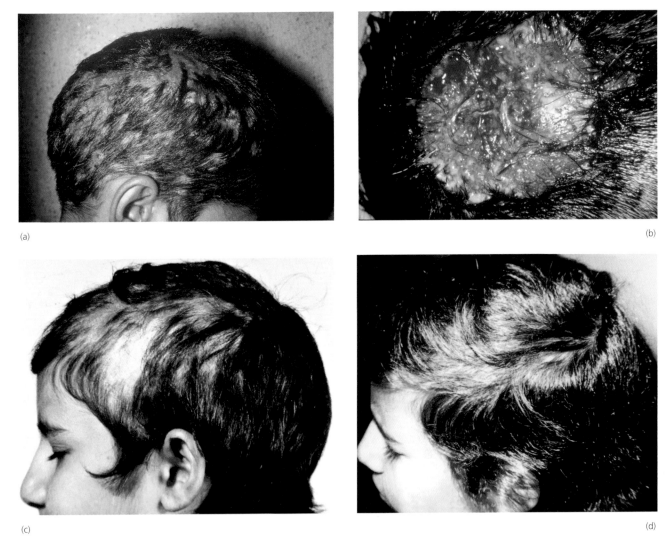

(a)

(b)

(c)

(d)

Figure 19.15 (a) Scalp fungus with alopecia. (b) Kerion. (c) Tinea capitis before treatment. (d) Tinea capitis after treatment.

Fungal infection

Trichophyton tonsurans causes a diffuse hair loss with broken hairs (Figure 19.15a). *Microsporum canis* or *Trichophyton mentagrophytes* may cause an acutely inflamed pustular mass containing few hairs – kerion (Figure 19.15b). Tinea capitis is rarely seen after puberty whereas tinea pedis, tinea cruris, and onychomycosis are usually seen in post-pubertal patients. For confirmation of a fungal lesion of the skin, scales are obtained from the border of a lesion. Hairs infected with a *Microsporum* species will fluoresce green when examined under a Wood's (long-wave UVL) lamp. In infections of the hair and nails a systemic antifungal agent, griseofulvin or terbinafine (unlicensed for children), is the treatment of choice (Figure 19.15c,d), but for skin infections alone a topical antifungal agent is usually adequate. In the latter group the imidazole derivatives such as clotrimazole, miconazole, and econazole have superseded the well-tried although cosmetically less acceptable benzoic acid compound (Whitfield's ointment).

Further reading

Harper J, Oranje A, Prose N. *Textbook of Paediatric Dermatology*, 2nd edn. Blackwell Publishing, Oxford, 2005.

CHAPTER 20

Febrile Convulsions

Bernard Valman

Northwick Park Hospital and Imperial College London, UK

OVERVIEW

- A febrile convulsion is a fit occurring in a child aged from 6 months to 5 years, precipitated by fever arising from infection outside the nervous system in a child who is otherwise neurologically normal.

- Convulsions with fever include any convulsion in a child of any age with fever of any cause. Among children who have convulsions with fever are those with pyogenic or viral meningitis, encephalitis, or cerebral palsy with intercurrent infections. Children who have a prolonged fit or who have not completely recovered within 1 hour should be suspected of having one of these conditions.

- Most of the fits that occur between the ages of 6 months and 5 years are simple febrile convulsions and have an excellent prognosis. If there is no fever the possibility of epilepsy should be considered (see Chapter 21).

Box 20.1 **Simple febrile convulsions**

All the following:
- Less than 20 minutes
- No focal features
- 6 months to 5 years
- No developmental or neurological abnormalities
- Not repeated in the same episode
- Complete recovery within 1 hour

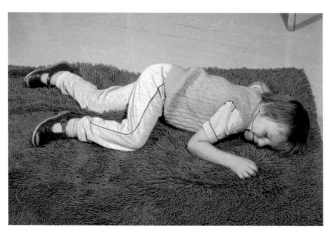

Figure 20.1 Child is placed in this position after a febrile convulsion.

Often fever is recognized only when a convulsion has already occurred. An abrupt rise in temperature rather than a high level is important. There may be a frightened cry followed by abrupt loss of consciousness with muscular rigidity, which form the tonic stage. Cessation of respiratory movements and incontinence of urine and faeces may occur during this stage, which usually lasts up to half a minute. The clonic stage which follows consists of repetitive movements of the limbs or face. By arbitrary definition, in simple febrile convulsions the fit lasts less than 20 minutes, there are no focal features, and the child is aged between 6 months and 5 years and has been developing normally before the convulsion (Box 20.1).

Rigors may occur in any acute febrile illness, but there is no loss of consciousness.

Emergency treatment

If the child has fever, he should be dressed in a single layer of clothes and covered with a sheet only. He should be nursed on his side or prone with his head to one side because vomiting with aspiration is a constant hazard (Figure 20.1).

If the child is still having a convulsion, buccal midazolam produces an effective blood concentration of anticonvulsant within 10 minutes and can be easily administered by parents or carers. Rectal diazepam is an alternative and can be administered by a convenient preparation which resembles a toothpaste tube (Stesolid) (Figure 20.2). This method of administration has become less acceptable recently. Early admission to hospital or transfer to the intensive care unit should be considered if a second dose of anticonvulsant is needed.

Some children who have had a first febrile convulsion should be admitted to hospital to exclude meningitis and to educate the parents, as many fear that their child is dying during the fit. Physical examination at this stage usually does not show a cause for the fever, but a specimen of urine should be examined in the laboratory to exclude infection and a dipstix test for glucose should be performed

ABC of One to Seven, 5th edition. Edited by B. Valman. © 2010 Blackwell Publishing, ISBN: 978-1-4051-8105-1.

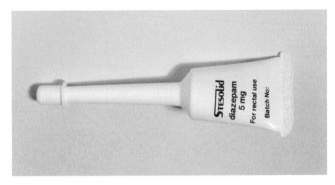

Figure 20.2 Rectal diazepam tube.

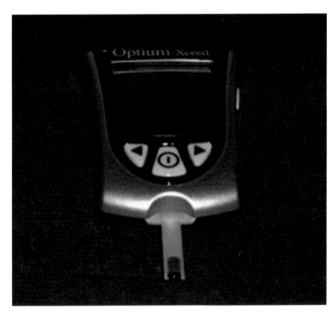

Figure 20.3 Blood check for glucose.

(Figure 20.3). Most of these children have a generalized viral infection with viraemia. A febrile convulsion may occur in roseola at the onset and 3 days later the rash appears. Occasionally, acute otitis media is present, in which case an antibiotic is indicated, but most children with febrile convulsions do not need an antibiotic.

Lumbar puncture

A lumbar puncture should be considered if the child is under 18 months old or any of the following are present:
1 Signs of meningism such as neck stiffness;
2 Drowsiness, irritability, or systemic illness;
3 Complex convulsion that contains any feature that does not conform to the definition of a simple convulsion.

The decision should be taken by an experienced doctor, who may decide on clinical grounds that lumbar puncture is unnecessary even in a younger child, but when in doubt the investigation should be performed. The doctor deciding not to undertake a lumbar puncture should review the patient personally within a few hours. If the convulsion is prolonged or has unusual features, there are features of raised intracranial pressure or a rash, a CT brain scan should be performed before the lumbar puncture. A child who has had severe

vomiting or is in coma must be examined by an experienced doctor and have a CT scan before lumbar puncture because of the risk of coning. Children less than 2 years of age may have meningitis with no neck stiffness or other specific signs.

An electroencephalogram (EEG) is not a guide to diagnosis, treatment, or prognosis.

Treatment

Management of fever

There is no evidence that antipyretic treatment influences the recurrence of febrile convulsions, but fever should be treated to promote the comfort of the child and to prevent dehydration. The child should be dressed in only one layer of clothing and should be covered with a sheet only. Paracetamol is the preferred antipyretic, and adequate fluid should be given. If the fever does not resolve with paracetamol, it is replaced by ibuprofen given alone.

Anticonvulsant drugs

Buccal midazolam or rectal diazepam should be used as soon as possible after the onset of the convulsion. The parents should be advised not to give it if the convulsion has stopped.

The only indications for long-term anticonvulsant prophylaxis after febrile convulsions are a prolonged initial convulsion or frequent recurrences. There is no evidence that the prophylactic use of anticonvulsant drugs in the minority of children who later develop epilepsy would have prevented it.

Immunization

As immunization against diphtheria, tetanus, pertussis, and poliomyelitis is given to children 2–4 months old, this schedule is usually completed before febrile convulsions occur. Babies having convulsions with fever aged less than 4 months should be assessed by a paediatrician. Children who have febrile convulsions before immunization against diphtheria, pertussis, pneumococcus, meningococcus, and tetanus because the immunization has been delayed should be immunized after their parents have been instructed about the management of fever and the use of buccal midazolam or rectal diazepam.

Measles, mumps, and rubella immunization should be given as usual to children who have had febrile convulsions, with advice about the management of fever to the parents. Buccal midazolam or rectal diazepam should be made available for use should a convulsion occur.

Prognosis

Unless there is clinical doubt about the child's current developmental or neurological state, parents should be told that prognosis for development is excellent. The risk of subsequent epilepsy after a single febrile convulsion with no complex features is about 1%. With each additional complex feature the risk of epilepsy rises to nearly 50% in children with three complex features by the age of 25 years (Box 20.2). Only about 1% of children with febrile convulsions are in this group.

Box 20.2 **Complex febrile convulsions**

- Lasting longer than 15 minutes
- Focal
- More than one on the same day
- First at age < 1 year
- Developmental or neurological abnormalities

Box 20.3 **Advice to parents – febrile convulsions**

Your child has had a febrile convulsion. We know it was a very frightening experience for you. You may have thought that your child was dead or dying, as many parents think that when they first see a febrile convulsion. Febrile convulsions are not as serious as they appear.

What is a febrile convulsion?
It is an attack brought on by fever in a child aged between 6 months and 5 years.

What is a convulsion?
A convulsion is an attack in which the child becomes unconscious and usually stiff, with jerking of the arms and legs. It is caused by unusual electrical activity of the brain. The words convulsion, fit, and seizure have the same meaning.

What shall I do if my child has another convulsion?
Lay him on his side, with his head on the same level or slightly lower than the body. Note the time. Do not try to force anything into his mouth. Do not slap or shake the child.

The hospital may give you medicine to insert into your child's mouth or for rubbing into the gums. This is called buccal midazolam. This treatment should stop the convulsion within 10 minutes. If it does not, take your child to the hospital. You may need to dial 999 to obtain an ambulance. Let your doctor know what has happened.

About 1 child in 30 will have had a febrile convulsion by the age of 5 years.

Is it epilepsy?
No. The word epilepsy is applied to fits without fever, usually in older children and adults.

Do febrile convulsions lead to epilepsy?
Rarely. Ninety-nine out of 100 children with febrile convulsions never have convulsions after they reach school age, and never have fits without fever.

Do febrile convulsions cause permanent brain damage?
Almost never. Very rarely a child who has a very prolonged febrile convulsion lasting half an hour or more may suffer permanent damage from it.

What starts febrile convulsions?
Any illness that causes a high temperature, usually a cold or other virus infection.

Will it happen again?
Three out of 10 children who have a febrile convulsion will have another one. The risk of having another febrile convulsion falls rapidly after the age of 3 years.

Does the child suffer discomfort or pain during a convulsion?
No. The child is unconscious and unaware of what is happening.

What shall I do if my child has fever?
You can take the child's temperature by placing the bulb of the thermometer under his armpit for 3 minutes with his arm held against his side. Keep him cool by putting on one layer of clothing and covering him by only a sheet. Give plenty of fluids to drink. Give children's paracetamol or ibuprofen to reduce the temperature. Repeat the dose every 4 hours until the temperature falls to normal, and then every 6 hours for the next 24 hours.

If the child seems ill or has ear ache or a sore throat, let your doctor see him in case any other treatment, such as an antibiotic, is needed. Antibiotics are not necessary for most children with fever caused by virus infections.

Is regular treatment with tablets or medicine necessary?
Usually not. The doctor will explain to you if your child needs regular medicine.

Adapted from a pamphlet produced by the Royal College of Paediatrics and Child Health.

The risk of having further febrile convulsions is about 30%. This risk increases in younger infants and is about 50% in infants aged less than 1 year at the time of their first convulsion. A history of febrile convulsions in a first degree relative is also associated with a risk of recurrence of about 50%. A complex convulsion or a family history of epilepsy is probably associated with an increase in the risk of further febrile convulsions.

Information for parents

Information for parents should include:
1 An explanation of the nature of febrile convulsions, including information about the prevalence and prognosis.
2 Instructions about the management of fever, the management of a convulsion, and the use of buccal midazolam or rectal diazepam.
3 Reassurance about the benign nature of febrile convulsions.
This advice should be given verbally and a supplementary leaflet is helpful (Box 20.3).

Further reading

Sadlir LG, Sheffer IE. Febrile seizures. *BMJ* 2007; **334**: 307–311.

CHAPTER 21

Epilepsy

Bernard Valman

Northwick Park Hospital and Imperial College London, UK

OVERVIEW

- Detailed observations of the episode by a witness are the most important guide to the diagnosis of a fit.

- Recurrent attacks with similar features are essential for the diagnosis of epilepsy.

- The attacks may cause changes of consciousness or mood or produce abnormal sensory, motor, or visceral symptoms or signs. These changes are caused by recurring excessive neuronal discharges in the brain, although the electroencephalogram (EEG) may be normal.

- Investigations are no substitute for a history taken carefully from a witness and the EEG should not be used to determine whether an episode is caused by a fit.

- Documented absence of fever is essential to exclude the more common problem of febrile convulsions (see Chapter 20).

- See Chapter 20 for emergency management of a fit.

Box 21.1 **Assessment of epilepsy**

- Developmental level
- Motor function
- Hearing
- Sight (including squint)
- Skin (tuberous sclerosis)

Tonic–clonic epilepsy

About 80% of children with epilepsy have tonic–clonic seizures. The child may appear irritable or show other unusual behaviour for a few minutes or even for hours before an attack. Sudden loss of consciousness occurs during the tonic phase, which lasts 20–30 seconds and is accompanied by temporary cessation of respiratory movements and central cyanosis. The clonic phase follows with jerking movement of limbs and face. The movements gradually stop and the child may sleep for a few minutes before waking, confused and irritable. The best prognosis occurs in older children and those who respond promptly to anticonvulsants. When epilepsy is secondary to a structural brain abnormality the prognosis may be less good.

Carbamazepine and sodium valproate are the commonly used drugs. Carbamazepine has special value in children with a structural brain abnormality. Sodium valproate should not be used in polytherapy in infants under the age of 3 years, or in liver disease as fatal hepatotoxicity may occur. The drug should also be stopped if there are prodromal signs of nausea, vomiting, anorexia, or lethargy. Anticonvulsants are given until 2–4 years have passed with no symptoms and then discontinued gradually over several months.

Over half of patients with idiopathic tonic–clonic epilepsy and normal EEG have no recurrence, and a similar good prognosis is found in over 75% of patients who have been free of seizures for 2 years.

Absence epilepsy

In typical absence attacks, episodes of altered consciousness lasting 10–15 seconds occur spontaneously and can be precipitated by hyperventilation. Typical absence attacks are rarely associated with developmental delay or a structural brain abnormality. There

---

The incidence of epilepsy is about 6 in 1000 schoolchildren whereas the incidence of children with febrile convulsions is about 30 in 1000 preschool children. A single seizure may need investigation but should not be called epilepsy and specific treatment is usually not indicated. When a second attack occurs within 1 month of the first, early treatment is mandatory and may influence long-term outcome.

Disability depends partly on the frequency and severity of the fits but also on the presence or absence of developmental delay, cerebral palsy, or defects in the special senses that would suggest a structural brain abnormality (Box 21.1). Most children with epilepsy attend normal schools, rarely have fits, and have no disability apart from the fits.

Epileptic syndromes can be divided into those with no established aetiology but where there is a probability of genetic origin (idiopathic or primary) and those with a known aetiology (symptomatic or secondary) in which a structural brain lesion is suspected or can be shown. Epileptic fits can be divided into generalized or partial seizures. Generalized seizures include tonic–clonic, absence, and myoclonic fits. Partial seizures include focal and temporal lobe fits.

ABC of One to Seven, 5th edition. Edited by B. Valman. © 2010 Blackwell Publishing, ISBN: 978-1-4051-8105-1.

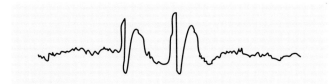

Figure 21.1 Electroencephalogram (EEG) in absence epilepsy.

is a typical EEG appearance (Figure 21.1) and the frequent attacks respond promptly to ethosuximide, sodium valproate, or lamotrigine introduced slowly. Treatment is continued for 2 years after the fits have been controlled.

Carbamazepine may exacerbate absence seizures, especially if the blood concentration is high.

Myoclonic epilepsy

Myoclonic epilepsy is caused by different brain insults; heredity may be implicated. Many of these children have developmental delay and some evidence of brain abnormality before the fits begin. The child may have a variety of seizures including:

1 Symmetrical synchronous flexion movements (myoclonic);
2 Brief loss of consciousness; or
3 Sudden head-dropping attacks (atonic–akinetic).

Infantile spasms are a form of myoclonic epilepsy which starts before the age of 1 year, has a characteristic EEG, and is treated with a course of prednisolone, or vigabatrin.

Perinatal asphyxia or acquired brain abnormality from any cause may have been present. Many of the children have developmental delay but the degree is variable. The EEG may remain normal long after the onset of the symptoms. Myoclonic epilepsy must be distinguished from absence epilepsy as treatment and prognosis are different.

Myoclonic seizures are often difficult to control with drugs. Sodium valproate is introduced gradually until the attacks cease or drowsiness occurs. Clobazam or lamotrigine are second line drugs.

Partial seizures

Partial seizures originate in specific areas of the brain and the symptoms depend on the site of the epileptic focus (Figure 21.2). A progressive space-occupying lesion is an extremely rare cause of this clinical picture. The most common variety of partial epilepsy in childhood is benign partial epilepsy of childhood where the focus is in the rolandic area. It usually starts between the ages of 7 and 10 years and attacks begin especially during sleep. Often they become generalized so that any generalized nocturnal convulsions may be due to this condition, which has a good prognosis. Consciousness is often retained but the child does not speak or swallow during the attack. There may be jerking of one side of the face with salivation, gurgling noises, and peculiar sensations affecting the tongue. Carbamazepine is extremely effective and most of the children are completely free of fits and then need no drugs shortly after puberty.

In contrast, the great variety of bizarre symptoms produced by fits originating in the temporal lobe makes diagnosis difficult and

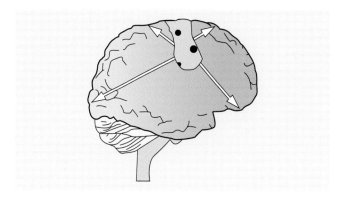

Figure 21.2 Partial seizures begin in a specific part of the brain.

attacks may be intractable despite anticonvulsants. There may be short episodes of emotional disturbance with the sudden onset of fear or rage, hallucinations of sight, sound, or smell, or visceral symptoms such as epigastric discomfort. A generalized tonic–clonic seizure may follow in some children. Carbamazepine is effective in about half of patients and is introduced slowly over several weeks to avoid drowsiness and ataxia.

When medical treatment has failed to control fits, referral to a paediatric neurology centre with advanced methods of investigation may allow the detection of a localized lesion which can be removed surgically.

Differential diagnosis

Breath-holding attacks

Convulsions need to be differentiated from breath-holding attacks, which usually begin at 9–18 months. Immediately after a frustrating or painful experience the child cries vigorously and then suddenly holds his breath, becomes cyanosed or pale, and in the most severe cases loses consciousness. Rarely, the limbs become rigid, and there may be a few clonic movements lasting a few seconds. The child takes a deep breath and regains consciousness immediately. The attacks diminish with age and there is no specific treatment. Mothers may be helped to manage these extremely frightening episodes by being told that the child will not die and that they should handle each attack consistently by putting the child down on his side.

Syncope

Syncope or a faint may occur at any age but is more usual in older children. While in the upright position the child appears very pale, becomes unsteady, and falls to the ground. There may be a precipitating factor such as standing in one position for a long time or being in a closed, hot room. Rarely, there may be a few clonic movements of the limbs but never a generalized convulsion and within a few minutes the child is perfectly normal again. He may say that he felt dizzy or unsteady at the beginning of the attack. Isolated episodes with obvious precipitating factors require no treatment.

Acute labyrinthitis

Acute labyrinthitis can cause episodes of dizziness. The child is frightened and may fall or vomit but does not lose consciousness.

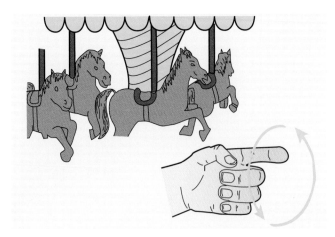

Figure 21.3 Acute labyrinthitis is a cause of vertigo.

If asked to draw the sensation in the air with a finger the child will describe a circular movement which suggests vertigo (Figure 21.3). This is caused by a viral infection affecting the balance mechanism of the inner ear which usually resolves within a few weeks, although attacks occasionally persist for longer.

Investigations

Investigations should be performed as outpatient procedures, keeping them to the minimum necessary for making a firm diagnosis and for excluding treatable causes. The specific tests will depend on the diagnosis made after taking the history and examining fasting plasma glucose, calcium, and urea concentrations. A dipstix test should be performed during a fit and if the result is abnormal blood is taken for a blood glucose estimation.

The EEG should not be used to determine whether a child has epilepsy; this is a clinical decision. About 50% of children with established epilepsy have a normal initial EEG. The EEG does not show whether the epilepsy is resolving or whether treatment can safely be stopped. However, the EEG may provide guidance on the type of epilepsy so that appropriate drugs are given, or it may show a unilateral lesion indicating the need for a brain scan by computed tomography (CT) or magnetic resonance imaging (MRI). Other indications for brain scan in children with fits are partial seizures (excluding benign rolandic epilepsy), poor medical control of fits, or developmental delay. Neuroimaging is not performed for children with primary generalized epilepsy (tonic–clonic seizures and typical absence epilepsy). Paediatricians should consider referring to a neurosurgeon those children whose fits are poorly controlled

medically. MRI is the ideal imaging technique in epilepsy but the long duration of the examination and the need for a general anaesthetic or deep sedation in young children results in limited availability. Lesions that may be detected are scars, tumours, and vascular and atrophic lesions as well as abnormalities of fetal brain development called focal cortical dysplasia.

Management

Measurements of blood or salivary anticonvulsant levels may help to prevent side effects and confirm compliance but the dosage must be determined mainly by the presence or absence of fits. Most children need only two doses of anticonvulsant each day and a single drug is the ideal. There is a prolonged remission in 75% of patients receiving monotherapy. If monotherapy is ineffective at the highest tolerated dose, a second drug should be used alone. The lowest dose that controls the seizures should be used. The effects on memory, attention, concentration, perception, and decision-making are twice as great with high than with low serum concentrations.

An adult must be present constantly at bath time and it is safer if the water is shallow (5.0–7.5 cm). Children with epilepsy should not ride a bicycle on the open road or swim unless there is an adult with them in the water. They should not climb ropes or high bars in a gymnasium. They can carry out all other activities. The school-teacher needs to know the child's diagnosis and be aware that most children with epilepsy have normal intelligence and should be expected to perform as well as their peers.

Learning difficulties may be a result of the effects of anticonvulsants, inattention caused by unrecognized fits, or underlying brain abnormality. Epilepsy is a family problem which can modify the lives of all members, and the parents will be worried about the child's prospects for future employment, driving a car, and marriage. They may believe, wrongly, that epilepsy is always associated with mental retardation. The doctor should tell the parents that the fits are not caused by a tumour and that a short fit does not injure the brain.

Further reading

National Institute for Clinical Excellence (NICE). *The Epilepsies: the Diagnosis and Management of the Epilepsies in Adults and Children in Primary and Secondary Care.* NICE Clinical Guidelines (CG 020). NICE, London, 2004. (www.nice.org.uk/cg020niceguideline)

Scottish Intercollegiate Guidelines Network. *Diagnosis and Management of Epilepsies in Children and Young People: a National Clinical Guideline.* Guideline 81. Scottish Intercollegiate Guidelines Network, Edinburgh, 2005. (www.sign.ac.uk)

CHAPTER 22

Recurrent Headache

Bernard Valman

Northwick Park Hospital and Imperial College London, UK

OVERVIEW

- Any acute illness with fever may cause headache, but if there is drowsiness, vomiting, photophobia, or neck stiffness an emergency lumbar puncture needs to be considered to exclude meningitis.

- Recurrent headaches are caused by migraine, emotional tension, or intracranial pathology. Emotional factors may precipitate attacks of migraine.

- Detailed physical examination is essential on the first visit, and reassessment is needed during the first 6 months after the onset of headaches to exclude a cerebral tumour that did not produce localizing symptoms or signs initially.

- The blood pressure should be measured and the fundi examined in every child with headache.

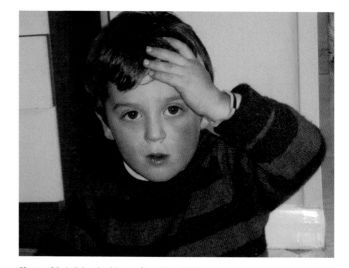

Figure 22.1 Take the history from the child.

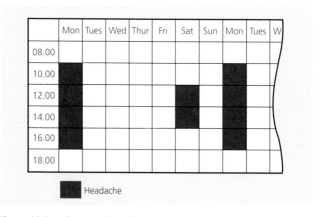

Figure 22.2 A diary may show the trigger factor.

Migraine

Migraine occurs in about 4% of children, and tension headaches probably have about the same prevalence. The pain of migraine is usually accompanied by nausea or vomiting and is relieved by sleep. There is often intolerance to light or noise and there may be pallor. The pain lasts for hours and there is complete freedom from pain between attacks. In about 20% of patients there is a hemicranial distribution of the pain, and in about another 20% there is vertigo or lightheadedness. Only about 5% of children with migraine have a visual aura. Migraine can occur at any age, but its apparent rarity under the age of 5 years may be because of children's difficulty in discussing their symptoms (Figure 22.1).

As 90% of children with migraine have parents or siblings with this condition, the absence of a family history throws some doubt on the diagnosis. However, 50% of all children have a family history of migraine, so the presence of this history is not helpful in diagnosis. Although they may have been called migraine, the details of the relatives' headaches may show that they have the features of emotional tension headaches.

Psychological stress is the most common trigger factor of attacks, and school is often implicated (Figure 22.2). The child may have

difficulty in keeping up with his peers or may fear impending examinations. Children are often seen by a doctor for the first time at the beginning of the new school year in September, but in other families the mother may cope until March or April. Some of these children are progressing well at school but pursue a very hectic life afterwards. The importance of specific foods is controversial but a mother may have observed that a particular food such as chocolate or cheese may consistently precipitate symptoms. This occurs in about 10% of children. Provided that only one type of food is

ABC of One to Seven, 5th edition. Edited by B. Valman. © 2010 Blackwell Publishing, ISBN: 978-1-4051-8105-1.

implicated, it can be excluded from the diet. Any more extensive alterations should be supervised by a paediatric dietitian. A head injury or acute upper respiratory tract infection may precipitate a series of attacks, but the importance of acute sinusitis either as a trigger factor in migraine or as a specific cause of recurrent headache has probably been exaggerated. Physical activity to exhaustion, mild hypoglycaemia as a result of missing a meal, excessive exposure to sun, or a lack of sleep may precipitate attacks in susceptible children.

Management

There are no abnormal signs on examination and no investigations are indicated when the diagnosis is clear clinically. The diagnosis is explained to the whole family, including the child, and it is pointed out that most children have exacerbations of 6 months' duration within 2–4 years after school-related exacerbations, followed by a remission which may last between 9 years and indefinitely. Avoidance of trigger factors may need exploration with the help of a school report and sometimes assessment by a psychologist. If the symptoms have been present for less than 6 months a further physical examination will be needed until enough time has elapsed to exclude an intracranial lesion. Although this possibility needs to be considered, it need not be transmitted to the parents, but many parents will be worried about the possibility of a tumour and the value of a normal examination can be emphasized.

Treatment of an acute attack is more likely to be effective if it is given early. A supply of paracetamol or ibuprofen should be kept at school as well as at home. If vomiting is a prominent early feature of attacks paracetamol can be given as a suppository or an antiemetic can be given early in an attack. If these treatments are not effective the child should be allowed to lie down in a darkened room for half an hour. If there is an attack once a week and the symptoms interfere with the child's life, regular continuous prophylactic treatment with propranolol or pizotifen may be recommended for 3 months by a paediatrician. Behaviour modification techniques have been successful where parents are motivated and staff with the necessary skills are available.

Emotional tension

The headache is often present every day, usually starting in the afternoon and continuing to the evening. It is described as an ache, tightness, or pressure affecting any part of the head (Figure 22.3). It is commonly frontal but may be felt in the temporal or occipital regions. Poor school attendance is common, with absence from school for weeks at a time. Evidence of environmental factors causing anxiety at school and at home should be sought, and there may be additional physical symptoms such as pain in the abdomen or limbs which complete the picture. There may be overt symptoms of psychiatric disturbance such as depression, disruptive behaviour in group activities, or destruction of property.

Repeated clenching or grinding of the teeth may cause tension headaches. The pain can be induced by clenching the teeth and pressing on the temporal muscles with the tips of the fingers. A plastic teeth mould made by a dentist may stop the teeth grinding.

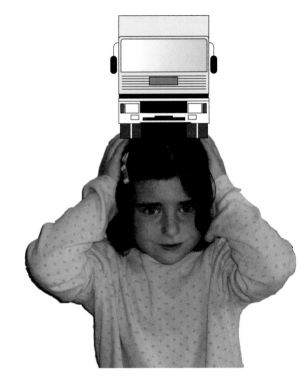

Figure 22.3 Sensation of pressure on the head.

Management

The absence of physical signs confirms the diagnosis and helps the family to accept it. If the headaches have been present for more than 6 months and there are no abnormal signs, the risk of a cerebral tumour is low. Specific investigations are seldom required, but a further assessment is needed to allow the parents to consider any further relevant factors, to discuss the school report with them, to plan further management, and to confirm the absence of abnormal physical signs if the history is short. Simple changes in the child's routine or environment or, occasionally, referral to a child psychiatrist, may be needed.

Intracranial lesions

Most intracranial lesions are cerebral tumours or vascular malformations, but a few are subdural haemorrhages or intracranial abscesses (Figure 22.4). These lesions do not produce a specific clinical picture, but there are some pointers that make the diagnosis more likely.

Abnormal physical signs are present in most children with intracranial lesions either when they are first seen or within 4 months of the onset of symptoms. About half of the children have papilloedema, and other common signs are disturbances in gait or hemiparesis.

Headache that wakes the child at night, is present on waking in the morning, or is aggravated by coughing suggests an intracranial lesion. The following are indications for referral to a paediatrician or paediatric neurologist, who will usually arrange computed tomography or magnetic resonance imaging of the brain as the first investigation:

1 Abnormal neurological signs during or after headache;
2 Fits with headache;

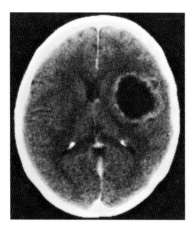

Figure 22.4 Computed tomography (CT) scan of intracranial lesion.

3 Nocturnal or early morning headache, especially if the history is shorter than 6 months or if the headaches are increasing in frequency or severity;

4 Recent school failure, change in behaviour – especially apathy or irritability – or failure to grow in height;

5 Change in quality or distribution of headache;

6 Extremely severe incapacitating headaches; and

7 Age less than 5 years.

Further reading

David RB, ed. *Child and Adolescent Neurology*, 2nd edn. Blackwells Publishing, Oxford, 2005.

CHAPTER 23

Poisoning

Bernard Valman

Northwick Park Hospital and Imperial College London, UK

OVERVIEW

- Accidental swallowing of drugs and household fluids is common among children, especially between the ages of 2 and 3 years.

- Most of them take trivial amounts of drugs, but every child must be assessed carefully to ensure that effective treatment is given when a potentially fatal dose has been swallowed.

- This chapter should be read with Chapter 26 on basic life support as the initial management is similar in all types of poisoning.

- A health visitor's report on the family may be helpful as the event may indicate a chaotic household or a non-accidental injury.

- Child-resistant containers have reduced the incidence of poisoning by tablets.

- Intentional overdose is a form of child abuse.

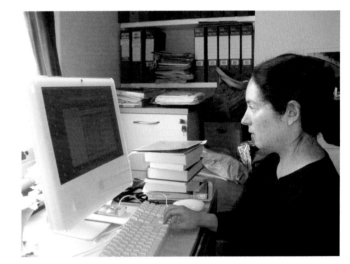

Figure 23.1 Access database for information.

This chapter gives an overview of the management of poisoning and either Toxbase or the UK National Poisons Information Service (see below) should be consulted where there is a doubt about the severity or management.

The name of the drug may be on the bottle, or the tablets may be identifiable from a computer program by Toxbase (Figure 23.1). The prescriber, hospital pharmacist, or the pharmacist who dispensed the tablets may be able to help. The time the drug was taken should be written in the clinical notes and whether any symptoms such as vomiting have occurred. The maximum amount of drug that could have been taken should be estimated. The original number of tablets in the bottle may be known. Usually the dispensing pharmacist knows the original number of tablets dispensed.

Non-poisons

Accidental ingestion of a substance known to be non-poisonous can be dealt with by reassurance alone. Antibiotics, vitamins, simple antacids, and oral contraceptives are not toxic. Homeopathic preparations are non-toxic but must be distinguished from herbal

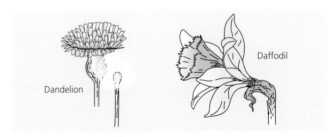

Figure 23.2 Non-poisonous plants.

preparations, which may contain enough active substances to cause symptoms.

Mild diarrhoea or vomiting may occur after the ingestion of plants, but most are non-toxic. Berries that are non-toxic include those of berberis, Chinese lantern, cotoneaster, hawthorn, mahonia, mountain ash (rowan), pyracantha, skimmia, and japonica. Most flowers are non-toxic – for example, antirrhinum, daffodil, bluebell, daisy, dandelion, fuschia, geranium, rose, violet, stock (Figure 23.2).

Bath soap, bubble bath, carpet cleaner, scouring powders, and dishwashing liquid are not toxic (Figure 23.3); however, dishwashing powders and tablets are highly alkaline (caustic). Innocuous

ABC of One to Seven, 5th edition. Edited by B. Valman. © 2010 Blackwell Publishing, ISBN: 978-1-4051-8105-1.

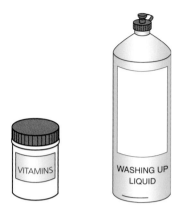

Figure 23.3 Non-poisonous substances.

Box 23.1 **Grading levels of consciousness**

- Fully conscious
- Drowsy but responds to verbal stimulation
- No response to verbal stimuli, localized response to painful stimuli
- No response to verbal stimuli, generalized response to painful stimuli
- No response to painful stimuli

---

water-based paints must be distinguished from oil-based paints in which the hydrocarbon solvents may be dangerous. Similarly, water-based glues are innocuous.

Nail varnish and nail varnish remover contain toxic solvents and perfumes contain alcohol, but the small amounts ingested are rarely enough to cause harm.

Anticoagulant rat baits such as warfarin are toxic only in massive or repeated doses, so a serious change in prothrombin time brought about by acute poisoning is very unusual. Many weedkillers and pesticides are relatively harmless in small amounts, but some can be toxic and it is important to find out the ingredients in each case.

Examination

Initially, protecting the airway, maintaining adequate ventilation and circulation is more important than making an exact diagnosis (Chapter 26). The level of consciousness is the most important single sign (Box 23.1). The frequency and depth of the respiratory movements are noted. Slow, shallow movements suggest impending respiratory arrest and the need for assisted ventilation. A raised pulse rate indicates shock and a low blood pressure shows that cardiac arrest is imminent.

Particles of tablets may be present in the mouth or vomit. The odour of paraffin (kerosene) may be present in the breath. Caustic or acid substances may cause burns on the lips and tongue and in the mouth. Deep sighing respiratory movements or a raised respiratory rate suggest salicylate poisoning, while tachycardia and dilated pupils are found in atropine poisoning. Opiates cause constriction of the pupils.

Children who have features of poisoning are usually admitted to hospital. Children who have taken poisons with delayed action should be admitted, even if they appear well when first seen. Poisons with delayed action include aspirin, iron, paracetamol, tricyclic antidepressants, paraquat, and Lomotil. Modified-release preparations may have a delayed effect.

General management

Prevention of absorption

Activated charcoal can absorb many poisons and reduce absorption. It should be given as soon as possible and may be effective if given up to an hour after ingestion – longer if modified-release drugs or antimuscarinic drugs have been given. It is relatively safe, but the airway should be protected if the child is drowsy. It can bind many poisons in the stomach, which reduces absorption, and repeated doses enhance the elimination of some drugs after they have been absorbed: carbamazepine, dapsone, phenobarbitone, quinine, and theophylline.

A specimen of vomit and of urine should be kept for possible analysis. Heparinized tubes should be used for collecting blood for salicylate estimation. The types of blood specimens required for estimating other poisons depend on the methods used in that laboratory.

Removal from the gastrointestinal tract

Gastric lavage is rarely performed as the benefit is usually outweighed by the risk of aspiration. It is only indicated if a life-threatening amount of drug has been taken within the previous hour, an anaesthetist is present to protect the airway, and the drug is not adsorbed by activated charcoal (see below). It is contraindicated if a corrosive substance or a petroleum distillate has been ingested.

Salicylate poisoning

The incidence of aspirin poisoning has fallen since the introduction of child-proof containers and the withdrawal of aspirin as an antipyretic in children. Vomiting and deep respiratory movements are early signs of salicylate poisoning and may mimic pneumonia, whereas drowsiness and coma are late features.

Methyl salicylate (oil of wintergreen) used as an embrocation in adults is dangerous, as only 4 mL may be fatal in infants. The child can usually tolerate a single acute ingestion of 100 mg/kg body weight of aspirin without serious effect. Blood concentration should be estimated 6 hours after ingestion and again several hours later to ensure that it is not continuing to rise. If the plasma salicylate concentration is over 300 mg/L (2.2 mmol/L) the child has moderate or severe poisoning. Intravenous fluids with frequent measurements of plasma salicylate, glucose, and electrolyte levels are needed to restore fluid and electrolyte balance and correct metabolic acidosis.

Barbiturates

Management after ingestion of barbiturates, benzodiazepines, and other sedative or hypnotic drugs is similar. As the smallest dose of barbiturates ingested is usually an adult dose the child must be admitted. The timing of the onset of symptoms depends on the type of barbiturate. Repeat estimations of the level of consciousness are essential for management and can be recorded on a chart (Box 23.1).

The child must be nursed prone or on his side to avoid aspirating vomit. Slow, shallow respiratory movements are signs of impending respiratory arrest. Hundred per cent oxygen can be given by mask or inflatable bag with mask, such as a Laerdal bag. An anaesthetist should be called immediately, and intubation and mechanical ventilation may be needed. Debris should be removed from the mouth with gauze swabs or by suction. Hypotension is treated initially by giving intravenous fluids to restore the central venous pressure.

Estimations of blood barbiturate concentrations do not help management but may be useful if there is doubt about the diagnosis. Clinical features are the best guide.

Paracetamol

The relatively small overdose of 150 mg/kg taken within 24 hours may cause severe hepatic necrosis. The early features are nausea and vomiting which resolve within 24 hours. Persistence beyond this time accompanied by right subcostal recession indicates hepatic necrosis. Liver damage is at the maximum 3–4 days after ingestion and may cause encephalopathy, haemorrhage, hypoglycaemia, and death. Liver necrosis is shown by jaundice, an enlarged tender liver, hypotension, and arrhythmias. Hypothermia, hyperthermia, hypoglycaemia, or metabolic acidosis may occur. Excitement and delirium may be followed by sudden coma, which may be fatal without specialized treatment. Despite minor initial symptoms, children who have ingested an overdose of paracetamol should be admitted to hospital urgently.

Activated charcoal should be considered if the amount of paracetamol ingested within the previous hour exceeds 150 mg/kg or 12 g, whichever is the smaller. Acetylcysteine given intravenously protects the liver if infused within 24 hours of ingesting paracetamol. It is most effective if given within 8 hours of ingestion of paracetamol. The risk of liver necrosis, and the need for acetylcysteine, can be assessed by a blood paracetamol level taken 4 hours after ingestion and compared with a paracetamol treatment graph (Figure 23.4). In remote areas, oral methionine can replace acetylcysteine as initial treatment.

Children receiving enzyme-inducing drugs such as carbamazepine and those who are malnourished may require treatment with acetylcysteine at lower blood levels.

Antidepressants

Tricyclic and related antidepressant drugs cause dry mouth, depression in the level of consciousness, hypotension, hypothermia, convulsions, respiratory failure, and arrhythmias. Drowsiness occurs within a few hours interrupted by periods of restlessness. Ataxia and tachycardia follow. If the child has taken more than 10 mg/kg body weight amitriptyline or imipramine then convulsions, coma, and respiratory depression occur rapidly. Hypotension and cardiac arrhythmias may occur and the child should be managed in the intensive care unit. Intravenous diazepam is effective in controlling convulsions.

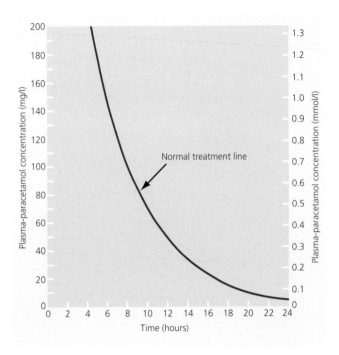

Figure 23.4 Treatment line for paracetamol poisoning. (Reproduced courtesy of the University of Wales College of Medicine Therapeutics and Toxicology Centre.)

Phenothiazines

The phenothiazines include chlorpromazine, which is used as a sedative, piperazine, used to treat threadworms, and perphenazine, prescribed as an antiemetic.

Drowsiness is common, even in therapeutic doses the effects of these drugs may resemble those of meningitis and there may be dyskinetic movements, including torticollis, facial grimacing, and abnormal eye movements. There may be symptoms similar to those seen in Parkinson's disease with muscular rigidity and tremor. Hypotension and hypothermia are common. The clinical features are similar to those of acute encephalitis or tetanus but there is no trismus.

Various cardiac arrhythmias may develop, and the electrocardiogram often shows prolongation of the Q–T interval and flattening of the T waves. The diagnosis may be confirmed by examining the urine for phenothiazine. Dyskinetic movements can be treated by intravenous benztropine or diazepam.

Iron

Toddlers may take their mother's iron tablets prescribed for pregnancy. Swallowing a large number may be followed by necrosis of the gastrointestinal wall and rapid absorption of iron. During the first few hours after ingestion there may be vomiting, haematemesis, and melaena, and severe abdominal pain accompanied by low blood pressure. After about 6–24 hours restlessness, convulsions, coma, and further haemorrhage may occur with metabolic acidosis and hepatic necrosis. All children who have ingested iron tablets should be admitted and kept in hospital for 48 hours because there may be a transient and deceptive improvement.

A blood concentration of over 90 mmol/L (500 pg/100 mL) suggests serious poisoning, but low levels cannot be considered safe as there may be rapid deposition of iron in the liver.

Blood should be taken for urgent serum iron estimation and grouping and cross-matching of blood. Gastric lavage, in the presence of an anaesthetist, and treatment with intravenous desferrioxamine should be considered.

Alcohol

Acute intoxication causes ataxia, dysarthria, and drowsiness. Children less than 10 years of age are particularly susceptible to the hypoglycaemic effects of alcohol, and any young child who has taken even a small wine glass of ordinary wine should therefore be admitted to hospital for frequent feeds containing glucose or a continuous intravenous infusion of 10% glucose. The blood glucose concentration must be monitored by dipstix readings at least every 3 hours for the first 24 hours.

In severe overdose taken intentionally by teenagers there may be coma, hypotension, and acidosis. The airway should be protected to avoid vomiting and fatal aspiration of gastric contents. Intravenous fluids and regular blood glucose measurements are needed.

Paraffin or turpentine

Although poisoning with paraffin is common, deaths, which are mainly due to respiratory complications, are rare. Turpentine is distilled from wood and differs chemically from paraffin but produces similar effects. Aspiration of paraffin into the lungs during ingestion or vomiting is the main danger, so emesis or gastric lavage should be avoided. There may be an increased respiratory rate, dyspnoea, and adventitious sounds, but extensive radiographical changes may be present with only slight symptoms. Radiological changes, which are usually bilateral, show patchy areas of consolidation in both lower lobes. Admission to hospital is always necessary as it may take 12 hours or more for the pulmonary features to appear.

Antihistamines

Some examples of antihistamines are chlorpheniramine, diphenhydramine, and promethazine. The clinical signs result from both

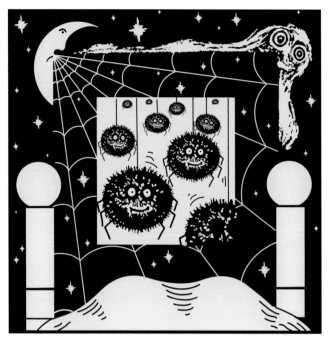

Figure 23.5 Antihistamines may cause hallucinations.

excitation and depression of the central nervous system. Drowsiness and headache may be followed by fixed dilated pupils, incoordination, hallucinations, excitement, and convulsions (Figure 23.5). Other effects include hypotension, tachycardia, and occasionally cardiac arrhythmias, respiratory depression, or hyperpyrexia. There is no specific antidote. Central nervous system excitation can be treated with diazepam.

Further reading

For information and advice in cases of poisoning contact the following centres:

UK National Poisons Information Service. Tel: 0870 600 6266 (24 hours). TOXBASE www .toxbase.org.

Help in identifying tablets or capsules may be obtained from regional medicines information centres.

BNF for Children 2007 (www. bnfc.org). Advisory line: 0151 252 5837 (www.dial.org.uk).

CHAPTER 24

Accidents

Bernard Valman

Northwick Park Hospital and Imperial College London, UK

OVERVIEW

• In 2005, in the UK, 251 children died as a result of injury or poisoning.

• Accidental injury is one of the biggest single causes of death in children over the age of 1 year.

• Every year over 2 million children are taken to hospital after an accident and about half of the accidents occur at home. The number of these accidents has fallen by 20% in the past 10 years.

• The largest number of injuries at home is due to falls especially in those under 5 years of age. Hot drinks causing scalds are more common than burns, but 18 children under 11 years died in house fires in 2005.

• In 2006 over 23,000 children were injured in road traffic accidents, 149 were killed, and 2828 were seriously injured.

About 1 child in every 4 attends the emergency department of the local hospital following an accident each year and large numbers of children are treated by their family doctors. Non-accidental injury and poisoning is dealt with in other chapters.

The word 'accident' implies that the event is not predictable or preventable, but prevention can be tackled by dividing the problem into factors concerning the child, the specific agent, and the circumstances. As accidents in the home form a large proportion of accidents, it may be possible to prevent a future death by pointing out possible hazards for children during a home visit. Health visitors, who routinely visit homes with young children, also play an important part in suggesting how the home can be made more safe. Accidents are also predictable from the developmental stage of the child, and doctors at clinics or surgeries can offer anticipatory advice tailored to the child.

Effect of social class and the long-term effects of accidents have been recognized. The social class gradient of accidental deaths is the steepest of all causes of death in childhood. Children in social class V are nine times more likely to die in a house fire than children in social class I and the difference is increasing. Prevention efforts should be directed towards the accidents experienced by socially deprived children.

About 10,000 children a year have some physical disability following an injury, but increasing attention is being paid to the psychological effects upon the child and the family.

Road accidents

Traffic is the most complicated environment that a child can experience. Children are unable to anticipate all types of hazards in traffic and do not know how to adapt to them.

Nearly 80% of children aged 5–9 years who are killed or seriously injured in road accidents are pedestrians, compared with 28% of road accident casualties of all ages. Parents should be taught that young children cannot judge traffic properly and need to be accompanied in busy traffic. Many accidents are caused by children dashing out into the road when vision is obstructed. Studies have shown that children conform to guidelines on safe behaviour better than adults, but adults' behaviour is often far from ideal, and they might influence children to copy them. The risk of an accident while crossing the road decreases from 5 to 11 years and the higher proportion of accidents in boys aged 5–7 than in girls may result from differences in behaviour, skills, and exposure during play. Children need to be aged at least 8 years before they can cross a quiet road safely, and at least 12 years for a busy road. Teaching and example are more important than any codes, which may be hard to understand and simply learnt by rote (Figure 24.1).

Government transport policy now encourages the reduction of car usage and environmental pollution as well as safety. A contribution to this is being made by trying to get children to school by public transport, by cycle, or by walking, and local authorities are encouraged to set up a 'Safer Routes to School' group in their area as a means to this end. Speed limits of 20 mph are now being introduced in some urban areas.

Cycling is also being encouraged by the organization Sustrans, which has established a national cycle network. Because about 70% of child cycle deaths are from head injuries, there is no

ABC of One to Seven, 5th edition. Edited by B. Valman. © 2010 Blackwell Publishing, ISBN: 978-1-4051-8105-1.

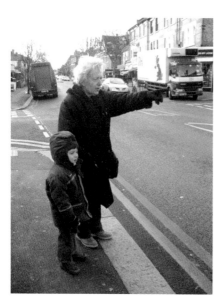

Figure 24.1 Teaching and example are more important than codes.

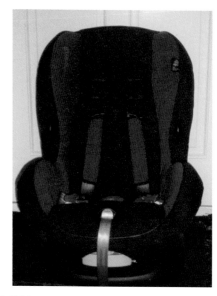

Figure 24.3 Child seat.

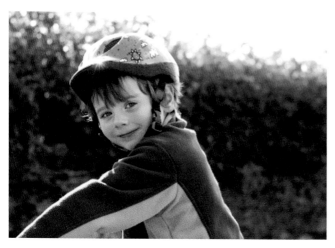

Figure 24.2 Cycle helmets are the best way to reduce cycle deaths.

doubt that the use of cycle helmets is the best way to reduce cycle deaths (Figure 24.2). The Child Accident Prevention Trust (CAPT) has a contract with a company to sell cycle helmets direct to schools at a reduced cost. The use of reflective clothing and lights at night and of satisfactory maintenance of bicycles is obviously important. Cycling proficiency tests have been established by the Royal Society for the Prevention of Accidents (RoSPA). Children under the age of 11 years should not cycle in traffic and still need adult supervision, because they do not have the skills to cope safely. Children should be encouraged to read the Highway Code for Young Users and attend a training course on road safety arranged by the local road safety officer.

Every year about 7000 children are injured and around 30 killed as car passengers on British roads. It is illegal for a passenger of any age to sit unrestrained in the front or in the back seat of a car. Appropriate restraints for different weights are as follows and the ages are given for guidance only:

- Babies up to 10 kg (6–8 months) rearward-facing infant carrier; but these should never be used on a passenger seat protected by an airbag.
- Toddler from 9 to 18 kg (9 months to 4 years). A child seat secured via its own frame by an adult seat belt or by its own special retention straps (Figure 24.3). Booster seats for toddlers and children from 15 to 25 kg (from 3–4 to 6 years) are also available, using an adult lap and diagonal belt.
- Children from 5–6 to 11 years (15–36 kg) can be restrained satisfactorily by a booster cushion using an adult lap and diagonal seat belt.
- Children 12 years or older should use an adult lap and diagonal belt. The centre seats in the rear of some cars now have lap and diagonal belts, which are better than lap belts alone.

Accidents in the home

Home accidents occur much more frequently than transport accidents, but because the forces involved are much less than those in road accidents the injuries produced are much less serious. Nevertheless, deaths from house fires are the second most common cause of death after road accidents. It is important to:

- *Prevent fires.* Safe smoking by adults; lock away matches; use child-resistant cigarette lighters; use fireguards.
- *Detect fires early.* Smoke detectors have been shown to be one of the most effective safety devices but need to be properly installed and maintained – for example, by replacing batteries when necessary (Figure 24.4). Carbon monoxide detectors are available.
- *Escape from fire.* Predetermined family fire escape plan taking fixed windows and double glazing into account.

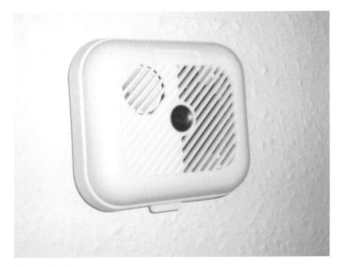

Figure 24.4 Smoke alarm.

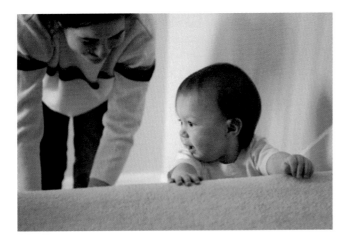

Figure 24.5 Supervision while climbing stairs.

Falls account for about 40% of toddler home accidents. Obviously, falls from a height cause more serious injuries than falls on the level. Falls downstairs can be prevented by the use of stair gates – preferably at the top and bottom of stairs, and the child should be supervised while learning how to climb up and down the stairs (Figure 24.5). Falls through horizontal or widely spaced banisters or balcony railings and out of windows have become less frequent following the introduction of new building regulations and better design. Baby walkers have been shown to be dangerous, producing falls down stairs or single steps, but also by being steered into fires. They are not recommended, but still remain very popular. Lacerations are a common form of injury, but the introduction of safety glazing by building regulations has reduced the size of this problem, although non-safety glazing still exists in older homes.

The principle of prevention in other household accidents is to keep the child away from the hazard. Medicines, matches, and household chemicals such as bleach and white spirit should be locked away. Pills and other dangerous substances should be in child-proof containers and never put in bottles or jars normally used for food or drink. Fires should be guarded, and parents need to be aware of how easily a child may be scalded by tipping over pans, kettles, and cups of hot liquid. The handles of pots should be turned away from the front of the cooker and electric kettles should have a short coiled lead. Knives and scissors should be kept out of sight in drawers. Peanuts are a common cause of choking in young children, and children may suffocate themselves with plastic bags left lying around. Encouragement to clear away toys after use will prevent tripping over them.

Playground equipment and use

The proper design and maintenance of playgrounds and their equipment is an important aspect of injury prevention for young children. Research has shown that impact-absorbent surfaces result in less serious injuries when a child falls on to them rather than on to concrete or asphalt, and local authorities are being strongly urged to replace the harder surfaces. Dangerous equipment such as long rocking horses have been replaced, but research has shown that monkey bars are a dangerous piece of more modern equipment. Slides built on the sides of mounds are safer than those with just metal supports. Play equipment is now being provided at public houses and shopping malls, and these need to be inspected as well as those provided by local authorities.

Swimming pools can be dangerous as a toddler can easily fall into a pool and be drowned. Children should be taught how to swim from the age of 5 years and not to dive into water that is less than 1.5 m (5 ft) deep.

Safety in other environments

Young children may visit farms, or may be part of a farmer's family. It is important that farmers should be aware of the special dangers presented by farm animals and equipment.

Making the environment as safe as is reasonably possible is probably a more effective means of injury and accident prevention than is the education of young children (Figure 24.6). However,

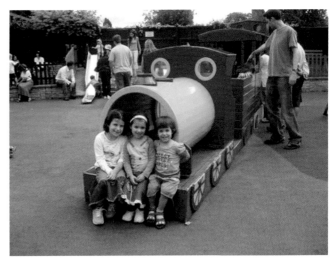

Figure 24.6 The environment should be safe.

people who design the environment and parents must recognize the importance of their role, and education is still important. The built environment can be designed for pedestrian-friendly streets, with humps in the roads to reduce the speed of traffic and safe routes to schools. The provision of play spaces and play areas offers interest and challenge as an alternative to playing in the streets or other more dangerous places.

A kitchen window that looks into the garden improves safety. The lower branches of trees can be removed to prevent the tree being climbed. An ice cream van on the opposite side of a busy road can also be dangerous. Railways and canals are hazards for children, and it is difficult to make every stretch of water and rail child-resistant by walls and fences. These may be damaged by vandals.

Doors to bathrooms and toilets should have handles that allow a bolted or locked door to be opened from the outside. Cooking stoves should be designed so that heated pots and pans as well as hot ovens are difficult for children to reach.

To be effective, protection must be provided for children of different ages and abilities. The toddler takes an overdose of medicine while exploring his environment, the 6-year-old dashes into the road without realizing the dangers, and the 12-year-old falls while climbing a tree. The very young cannot be taught how to avoid these dangers and therefore must be protected from them. As children grow older their parents and teachers can teach them how to cope with dangerous situations such as roads, warn them of other dangers, and help them to assess what is a reasonable risk.

Further reading

Child Accident Prevention Trust, 22–26 Farringdon Lane, London, EC1R 3AJ. Tel: 020 7608 3828. www.capt.org.uk. Provides booklets, fact sheets, and advice.

CHAPTER 25

Severely Ill Children

Bernard Valman

Northwick Park Hospital and Imperial College London, UK

OVERVIEW

- This chapter should be read with those on basic life support (Chapter 26) and fever (Chapter 27).

- The order of priorities is to provide basic life support, consider the probable diagnoses, and provide appropriate treatment.

- There is no precise definition of a severely ill child, but there are several conditions that need urgent treatment if the child is to survive. In most cases the treatment will be started in the community, ambulance, or the emergency department.

- A glance at a child will show that he is desperately ill and that a rapid history and examination are needed.

- The time of onset and duration of the symptoms should be noted. Questions must include the presence of rash, occurrence of diarrhoea, vomiting, cough, or fast breathing. The child may be receiving drugs or have had access to tablets or household fluids. Recent loss of weight should be noted.

Box 25.1 **SAFE approach**

Shout for help
Approach with care
Free from danger
Evaluate ABC

Box 25.2 **ABC**

Level of consciousness
Airway
Breathing
Circulation

Table 25.1 Normal heart rate by age at rest (for respiratory rate see Table 25.5).

Age (years)	Heart rate (beats/minute)
<1	110–160
1–5	95–140
5–12	80–120
>12	60–100

Immediate management

Rapid assessment, calling for assistance, and the initiation of management should take place within 1 minute (Box 25.1). The response to calling the child's name or pinching a digit indicates the level of consciousness (Box 25.2). Ensuring a clear airway, adequate ventilation, and circulation are the priorities. As vomiting and aspiration are constant hazards, a suction pump with a catheter of adequate bore should be kept next to the patient and turned on before the examination begins. If the child is not breathing or the respiratory rate is slow (Table 25.1), the airway may be blocked by the tongue falling back to obstruct the pharynx. An attempt should be made to open the airway using the chin lift manoeuvre (Figures 25.1 and 25.2). One hundred per cent oxygen is given with a mask. If there is a possibility of a foreign body see p. 18. Movements of the chest, breath sounds on auscultation, and the sensation of breath on the rescuer's face held near the child indicate effective treatment. If attempts at airway opening are not effective, mouth to mouth exhaled breathing is given, followed by ventilation

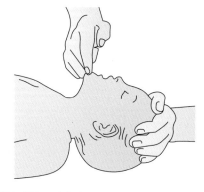

Figure 25.1 Chin lift in an infant.

ABC of One to Seven, 5th edition. Edited by B. Valman. © 2010 Blackwell Publishing, ISBN: 978-1-4051-8105-1.

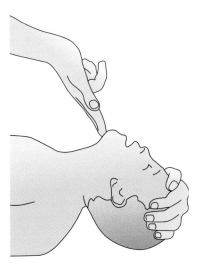

Figure 25.2 Chin lift in a child.

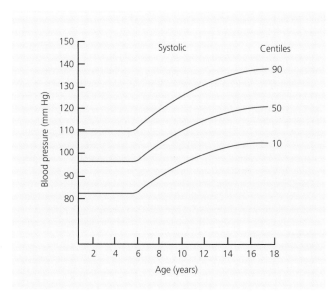

Figure 25.4 Normal range of blood pressure.

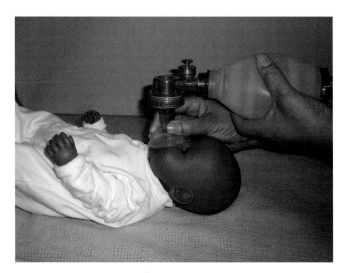

Figure 25.3 Ventilation with inflatable bag and mask.

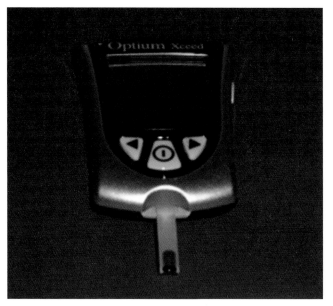

Figure 25.5 Glucometer.

using an inflatable bag and mask with oxygen (Figure 25.3) and later intubation and artificial ventilation.

Absence of a central pulse for 10 seconds or a pulse rate less than 60 per minute (Table 25.1) are indications for cardiac compression. The carotid pulse is used in infants and brachial or femoral pulses in children. A heart rate more than 160 beats/minute in infants and 140 beats/minute in children indicates potential circulatory failure and the need for urgent intravenous fluid (Table 25.1). Although a rise in temperature may be associated with the rise in heart rate, it must be assumed that a heart rate of this magnitude is potentially lethal and immediate transfer to a high dependency or an intensive care unit is indicated. Absent peripheral pulses and weak carotid pulses are other indicators of severe shock but a low blood pressure is an unreliable sign and may only occur terminally (Figure 25.4). Severe compromise of the peripheral circulation and the need for urgent intravenous fluids is also shown by a difference between the peripheral and core temperatures of more than 2°C or a capillary refill time of more than 3 seconds. If the ambient temperature is

normal, pressure on a digit for 5 seconds is normally followed by return of the normal colour within 3 seconds.

Blood glucose test

A glucose dipstix test with a glucometer (Figure 25.5) should be carried out before the physical examination. If the blood glucose concentration is more than 11 mmol/L (200 mg/100 ml) the child probably has diabetic ketoacidosis. If the blood glucose value is below 2.5 mmol/L (45 mg/100 ml) hypoglycaemia resulting from insulin overdose, salicylate poisoning, alcohol ingestion, or an inborn error of fatty acid, amino acid, or organic acid metabolism should be considered.

Table 25.2 Urgent investigations.

Diabetes mellitus	Glucometer, plasma glucose, urea, sodium, potassium, bicarbonate
Head injury	Computed tomograph of the brain
Poisons (including lead)	Glucometer, analysis of vomitus, urine, blood
Septicaemia with meningitis	Blood culture, lumbar puncture or osteomyelitis
Gastroenteritis	Glucometer, plasma sodium, potassium, bicarbonate
Continuous convulsions	Glucometer, plasma calcium and sodium
Upper airway obstruction	
Bronchopneumonia	Chest radiograph
Bronchiolitis	Chest radiograph
Paroxysmal tachycardia	Electrocardiograph
Peritonitis	Radiographs of abdomen, ultrasound

Table 25.3 Signs of dehydration and volumes of deficit.

Signs	Percentage dehydration	Deficit (mL/kg body weight)
Thirst	<5%	30
Reduced skin turgor	5%	50
Sunken eyes		
Depressed fontanelle		
Oliguria		
Tachycardia	8%	80
Apathy		
Cold limbs		
Capillary refill time 3 seconds or more		

Box 25.3 **Causes of drowsiness or loss of consciousness**

- Fit
- Head injury
- Drugs
- Septicaemia? with meningitis

Table 25.4 Maintenance water requirements for 24 hours.

Age (years)	Amount (mL/kg body weight)
0–2	80
3–5	70
6–9	60
10–14	50
>15	30

Urgent investigations

After the history has been taken and physical examination performed, urgent investigations are performed according to the predominant feature or probable diagnosis (Table 25.2).

Drowsiness and loss of consciousness

If the child is drowsy or unconscious the parents should be questioned about the possibility of a recent fit, head injury, or drug ingestion (Chapter 23) (Box 25.3). If there is any doubt, plasma salicylate and barbiturate concentrations may need to be measured. Septicaemia does not produce specific signs, just a generally ill child, and there may be associated meningitis. Neck stiffness is often absent in infants with meningitis who are less than 2 years old. Urine should be kept for drug analysis.

If aspiration of gastric contents is being considered, an anaesthetist should be consulted and be present during the procedure to prevent inhalation of gastric contents.

A severely dehydrated child has sunken eyes, a dry tongue, and inelastic skin and has usually not passed urine for several hours. The extent of recent weight loss may be known.

Acute gastroenteritis

Acute gastroenteritis should be considered if there has been diarrhoea with or without vomiting. Vomiting may be the only

symptom during the first 24 hours of gastroenteritis caused by rotavirus, but the possibility of another cause, such as intestinal obstruction, should be considered if vomiting is the only symptom. Infants may become severely ill before passing many loose stools as there may be pooling of fluid in the gut. Rectal examination may produce a large amount of fluid stool.

Clinical signs may be helpful in assessing the severity of dehydration (Table 25.3) and this may be confirmed by measured weight loss. In a severely dehydrated infant 20 mL 0.9% sodium chloride solution for each kilogram of body weight should be given intravenously by syringe, using any large vein but preferably not the femoral vein.

The aim is to complete rehydration 24 hours after admission but if hypernatraemia is present rehydration is completed over 48 hours. The total volume required is the amount needed to make up the deficit added to the maintenance volumes (Tables 25.3 and 25.4). The initial infusion is 0.45% sodium chloride solution with 5% glucose solution. The results of electrolyte estimations carried out on admission should be available within an hour and if the plasma potassium is not raised, a supplement of 10 mmol potassium chloride should be included in each 500 mL bag of fluid. Infusion solutions containing potassium should be supplied ready-mixed from the pharmacy, as fatal potassium overdose can occur if the solution is not thoroughly mixed. During the first 24 hours of admission no fluids or solids are given orally. The next day maintenance volumes of fluid are given as oral glucose electrolyte mixture, alternating with a full-strength cows' milk preparation and the addition of fruit and vegetable purée. The following day a normal diet is given. The frequency of the stools falls with effective treatment, but the consistency of the stools remains abnormal for about a week. If frequent stools return or the consistency does not become normal within 10 days, the possibility of cows' milk protein intolerance should be considered (see p. 40).

Diabetic ketoacidosis

If diabetic ketoacidosis is present (blood glucose concentration over 11 mmol/L (200 mg/100 ml)) intravenous 0.9% sodium chloride solution is needed urgently and intravenous insulin is started 1 hour later. A senior member of the paediatric unit should be informed immediately but the intravenous fluid should be started in the emergency department. There are often deep, frequent respiratory movements due to metabolic acidosis.

Plasma glucose, potassium, sodium, and urea concentrations and pH should be estimated on admission and at least at 2 and 6 hours after the beginning of treatment. Plasma glucose and urinary ketones should be measured hourly.

The initial intravenous fluid is 0.9% sodium chloride solution, which is given at a rate of 10–20 mL/kg body weight in the first 30 minutes. The aim is to rehydrate the child over 48 hours with the deficit added to the maintenance volumes (Tables 25.3 and 25.4). Many units no longer use sodium bicarbonate solution as the metabolic acidosis is corrected without it. Provided that the plasma potassium concentration is not raised, supplementary potassium chloride is given in a ready-mixed bag from the pharmacy (see above). In the pharmacy, 20 mmol of potassium chloride is added to every 500 mL bag of fluid. Oral potassium supplements are given when the child can drink. When the blood glucose concentration falls below 15 mmol/L (270 mg/100 ml) the fluid is changed to 0.45% sodium chloride with 5% glucose solution and supplementary potassium. Usually, 0.9% sodium chloride solution is given for about 6 hours before the change of solutions.

Insulin for initial treatment should always be the short-acting type of soluble insulin, given as a continuous intravenous infusion using a syringe pump. Every hour 0.05–0.1 units/kg are given. When the child is able to eat solid food (usually the next day) a subcutaneous injection of a short-acting insulin is given before each of the three main meals.

Headache or decreasing level of consciousness are features of significant cerebral oedema and intravenous mannitol should be considered.

Acute gastric dilatation is common in severe ketosis, and the stomach contents should be aspirated, in the presence of an anaesthetist, in a drowsy or unconscious patient to avoid aspiration pneumonia.

Convulsions

Convulsions associated with fever occur in 3% of children aged 6 months to 5 years. Often there is no warning and the fever is not obvious to the mother. The child should be dressed in a single layer of clothes and he should be covered with a sheet. If the convulsions persist or start again, buccal midazolam or rectal diazepam (Stesolid) at a dosage of 0.5 mg/kg is given. If the convulsions do not stop within 10 minutes, the duty anaesthetist should be present while another drug is given intravenously.

Early transfer to the intensive care unit should be considered if a second dose of anticonvulsant is needed. Intravenous diazepam is extremely effective but it has been associated with respiratory arrest, especially when the patient has previously received barbiturate or the drug has been given too quickly. Standard solutions of diazepam cannot be diluted, which may lead to inaccuracy in measuring small doses. Inserting and holding the needle in the vein of a convulsing, fat toddler is often a difficult task. Intravenous diazepam is best used only by those experienced in intubating infants.

Stridor

Stridor with drowsiness is a dangerous combination of signs, and the duty anaesthetist should be called to the child immediately. Cyanosis is a terminal sign in these infants. The throat and mouth must not be examined nor a throat swab taken except by a skilled anaesthetist prepared to perform immediate intubation or tracheostomy if necessary. Although most patients with stridor have laryngitis, a few have epiglottitis or an inhaled foreign body, and an examination of the throat in these last two conditions may cause complete obstruction of the respiratory tract followed by cardiac arrest. The child should be admitted to the intensive care unit or taken direct to the operating theatre, as urgent intubation by a skilled anaesthetist may be required.

Raised respiratory rate

A raised respiratory rate at rest suggests pneumonia or peritonitis (Figure 25.6). The upper limit for the normal respiratory rate at rest varies with age (Table 25.5). Pneumonia may make the child extremely ill because of the associated septicaemia. Pneumonia causes the alae nasi to move actively and there may be a cough, fever, and added sounds in the chest.

Infants with bronchiolitis may deteriorate suddenly and a rasping cough and recession of the chest wall may be the main features. If there was choking just before the dyspnoea began the possibility of an inhaled foreign body must be considered. When an enlarged liver accompanies a raised respiratory rate congestive cardiac failure is present. If there is no cardiac murmur, paroxysmal supraventricular tachycardia should be considered.

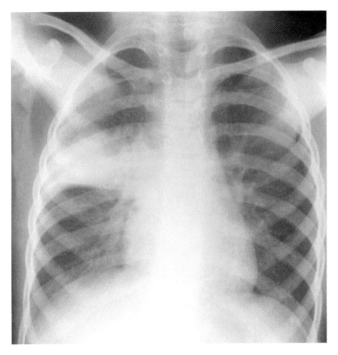

Figure 25.6 Pneumonia.

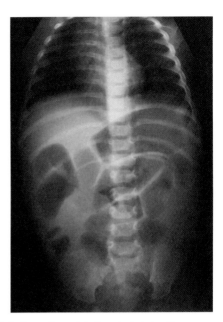

Figure 25.7 Supine radiograph in intestinal obstruction.

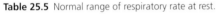

Table 25.5 Normal range of respiratory rate at rest.

Age (years)	Respiratory rate/minute
<0.2	35–60
0.2–1.0	30–40
1–2	30–35
2–5	25–30
5–12	20–25

Abdominal tenderness

Generalized abdominal tenderness suggests peritonitis, which may be caused by perforation of the appendix or of the small gut after intestinal obstruction. An obstructed inguinal hernia is a form of intestinal obstruction that is easily missed. In suspected intestinal obstruction urgent radiographs should be taken in the supine and erect positions to show fluid levels in distended loops of small gut (Figures 25.7 and 25.8). Fluid levels are also found in children with gastroenteritis but are present in the large gut as well as the small intestine. If the patient cannot stand erect similar information can be obtained from radiographs taken using a horizontal beam with the patient lying on his side.

Rash

If there is a purpuric rash that does not disappear when pressure is applied and which is not raised above the surface of the skin,

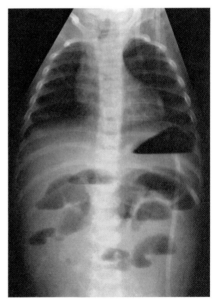

Figure 25.8 Erect radiograph in intestinal obstruction.

a presumptive diagnosis of meningococcal septicaemia should be made (Figure 25.9).

Blood should be taken for culture, and, using the same needle in the vein, benzylpenicillin is given slowly intravenously. The dose is 600 mg for children aged 1–9 years and 300 mg for younger children. If facilities for taking blood are not immediately available the penicillin should be given by the intramuscular route. Children may die within a few hours of the onset of this disease and urgent treatment is necessary.

In 10–20% of children with meningococcal disease the rash consists of large macules without purpura.

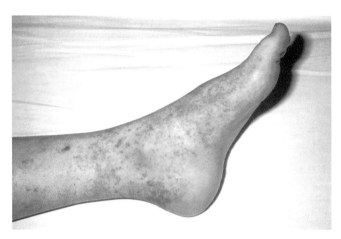

Figure 25.9 Rash of meningococcal septicaemia.

Further reading

BNF for children. BMJ Publishing Group, 2007 (www.bnf.org).

British Society for Paediatric Endocrinology and Diabetes (BSPED). Diabetic Ketoacidosis Guidelines (www.BSPED.org.uk).

Mackway-Jones K, Molyneux E, Phillips B. Wieteska S, eds. *Advanced Paediatric Life Support*, 4th edn. Blackwell Publishing, Oxford, 2005.

National Institute for Clinical Excellence (NICE). *Feverish Illness in Children.* NICE Clinical Guideline 47. NICE, 2007.

CHAPTER 26

Basic Life Support in the Community

Bernard Valman

Northwick Park Hospital and Imperial College London, UK

OVERVIEW

• Basic life support should be given immediately whenever an infant or child stops breathing, even if no specialized equipment is available. It may be life saving.

• An approved sequence of actions should be taken (Box 26.1).

Box 26.1 **Sequence of basic life support**

• Call for help
• Check environment is safe
• Assess condition
• Airway
• Breathing
• Circulation

Assessment of condition

The level of consciousness of the infant should be quickly assessed by gentle pressure on the shoulders or limbs together with a verbal command. Even young infants may open their eyes or move in response to sound if they are not unconscious. Young infants should not be shaken as this may result in brain haemorrhage from trauma caused by the mobile brain hitting the inside of the skull. If the infant is not responsive, then the ABC of basic life support should be followed.

Airway

The rescuer can assess whether the infant is breathing by placing their face closely above the infant's face in order to look, listen, and feel for breathing and chest movement. If the infant is not breathing, the head of the infant should be maintained in the neutral position (head in line with body) by gentle pressure with one of the rescuer's hands on the forehead and chin lift or jaw thrust under the angles of the mandible with the other hand (Figures 26.1 and 26.2). Flexion or overextension of the neck of an infant may cause obstruction of the upper airway by the tongue blocking the pharynx. Attempts to improve an obstructed airway with the rescuer's finger are not recommended and may be dangerous.

Breathing

The rescuer should give five exhaled breaths, each lasting approximately 1 second, into the infant's mouth or mouth and nose. The chest of the infant should be seen to expand with each breath or

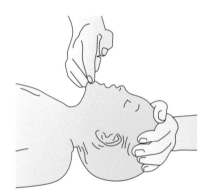

Figure 26.1 Chin lift in infant.

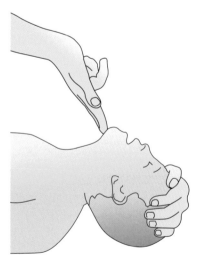

Figure 26.2 Chin lift in child.

ABC of One to Seven, 5th edition. Edited by B. Valman. © 2010 Blackwell Publishing, ISBN: 978-1-4051-8105-1.

else the airway is not clear and airway opening manoeuvres should be repeated.

Circulation

After five initial breaths, the pulse should be assessed by palpation of the brachial artery in the medial aspect of the antecubital fossa or femoral artery in the groin. The carotid artery is difficult to palpate in infants because the neck is often short and fat. If the pulse is absent or less than 60 beats/minute as assessed over 10 seconds, then external cardiac compressions should be commenced.

External cardiac compression

Cardiac compressions should be applied with the child lying flat on the back on a firm surface. There are two methods of compressions in small infants:

- Hands encircling the thorax with the thumbs compressing the sternum one finger breadth below an imaginary line drawn between the nipples (Figure 26.3). This method is only possible in very small infants and is difficult for a lone rescuer to perform along with mouth to mouth with or without nose breaths.
- Two-finger technique with the ball (not tips) of two fingers compressing the chest with the fingers again placed one finger breadth below the imaginary line between the nipples (Figure 26.4).

Whichever method is used, the chest should be compressed by about one-third depth in order to propel blood to the coronary arteries.

For children, the heal of the hand is placed over the lower third of the sternum which is depressed to about one-third of the depth of the chest (Figure 26.5).

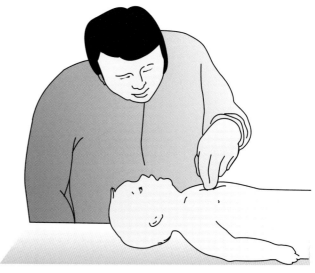

Figure 26.4 Alternative external cardiac compression in infant.

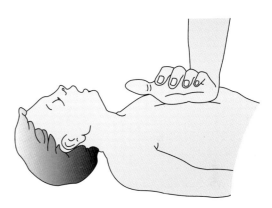

Figure 26.5 Chest compressions in a child.

Continue cardiopulmonary resuscitation

Cardiopulmonary resuscitation (CPR) should be continued with a ratio of 15 chest compressions to 2 breaths for approximately 1 minute before reassessment. The compression rate is 100 per minute. It is not necessary to simulate the heart rate of a normally breathing infant and indeed it may not be possible to do so in an effective manner. The rescuer should continue CPR until the emergency services arrive and take over resuscitation or if no help has arrived within a few minutes, the infant should be carried quickly to where help can be summoned.

Further reading

Mackway-Jones K, Molyneux E, Phillips B. Wieteska S, eds. *Advanced Paediatric Life Support*, 4th edn. Blackwell Publishing, Oxford, 2005.

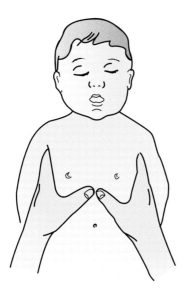

Figure 26.3 External cardiac compression in infant.

CHAPTER 27

The Child with Fever

Bernard Valman

Northwick Park Hospital and Imperial College London, UK

There should be an assessment of any life-threatening features including compromise of the airway, breathing, circulation, or decreased level of consciousness.

The risk factors below should be reviewed and the source of the fever should be sought.

Detection

The temperature should be measured by an electronic thermometer in the axilla or an infrared tympanic thermometer in the ear. The normal axillary temperature is 37.0°C (98.4°Fahrenheit). The normal tympanic membrane temperature is about 37.5°C (99.5°F). If the temperature is 0.6°C (1°F) above these levels, the child has a fever.

Assessment of risk

Table 27.1 provides a method for the assessment of the risk of a serious illness and the indications for immediate management

ABC of One to Seven, 5th edition. Edited by B. Valman. © 2010 Blackwell Publishing, ISBN: 978-1-4051-8105-1.

while the specific diagnosis of the cause of the fever is being sought.

Health care professionals receiving information by telephone should seek to establish the presence or absence of as many of the features in Table 27.1 as possible and children who need an urgent face-to-face assessment should be seen within 2 hours.

In primary care the following should be measured and recorded: heart rate, respiratory rate, and capillary refill time (CRT).

If no specific diagnosis has been reached, a safety net for parents should be provided if any intermediate risk factors are present. The safety net should be one of the following:

- Referral to specialist paediatric care for further assessment;
- Liaising with other health care providers, including out of hour providers, to ensure direct access for the patient for further assessment;
- Arranging further follow-up at a certain time and place;
- Providing the carer with verbal and written information on warning symptoms and how further health care can be accessed.

Immediate investigations and management

Infants less than 3 months old or in the high-risk group

If the temperature is 38°C or greater, the infant should be admitted to hospital immediately and the following should be measured: temperature, heart rate, and respiratory rate.

Children older than 3 months
Low risk group

Children with fever without apparent cause and have no features of serious illness, but need an urgent face to face assessment should be seen within 2 hours. After a history and examination have been performed, they should have urine collected by clean catch and tested for infection. They should also be assessed for signs of pneumonia.

Intermediate risk group

Children with fever without apparent cause and have one or more intermediate risk features should be seen in the paediatric ambulatory care, day-care unit, or emergency department urgently:

- Urine should be collected by clean catch and tested for infection;

Table 27.1 Traffic light system for identifying likelihood of serious illness.

	Green – low risk	Amber – intermediate risk	Red – high risk
Colour	• Normal colour of skin, lips and tongue	• Pallor reported by parent/carer	• Pale/mottled/ashen/blue
Activity	• Responds normally to social cues • Content/smiles • Stays awake or awakens quickly • Strong normal cry/not crying	• Not responding normally to social cues • Wakes only with prolonged stimulation • Decreased activity • No smile	• No response to social cues • Appears ill to a healthcare professional • Unable to rouse or if roused does not stay awake • Weak, high-pitched or continuous cry

Respiratory		• Nasal flaring
		• Tachypnoea:
		  – RR > 50 breaths/minute age 6–12 months
		  – RR > 40 breaths/minute age > 12 months
		• Oxygen saturation ≤ 95% in air
		• Crackles
			• Grunting
			• Tachypnoea:
			  – RR > 60 breaths/minute
			• Moderate or severe chest indrawing

Hydration	• Normal skin and eyes • Moist mucous membranes	• Dry mucous membrane • Poor feeding in infants • CRT ≥ 3 seconds • Reduced urine output	• Reduced skin turgor
Other	• None of the amber or red symptoms or signs	• Fever for ≥ 5 days • Swelling of a limb or joint • Non-weight bearing/not using an extremity • A new lump > 2 cm	• Age 0–3 months, temperature ≥ 38°c • Age 3–6 months, temperature ≥ 39°c • Non-blanching rash • Bulging fontanelle • Neck stiffness • Status epilepticus • Focal neurological signs • Focal seizures • Bile-stained vomiting

CRT, capillary refill time; RR, respiratory rate.

• Further investigations (e.g. C-reactive protein, white blood cell count, blood cultures) should be performed unless deemed unnecessary by an experienced paediatrician;
• Lumbar puncture should be considered in children less than 1 year of age;
• Chest radiograph for children with fever more than 39°C and white cell count more than 20×10^9/L.

High risk group

Children with fever without apparent cause presenting with one or more features of high risk should be transferred immediately to the hospital emergency unit or admitted directly to hospital (Chapter 25).

The following investigations should be performed:
• Blood culture;
• Full blood count;
• Urine testing for infection;
• C-reactive protein.

The following investigations should also be considered as guided by clinical assessment:
• Lumbar puncture in children of all ages if not contraindicated;
• Chest radiograph irrespective of temperature and white cell count;
• Blood glucose and serum electrolytes.

Features of specific illnesses

For the features of specific illnesses see Chapter 25 (see p. 94). A summary is given in Table 27.2.

Management of children in high or intermediate risk groups

Children with fever and shock should receive an immediate intravenous bolus of 20 mL 0.9% sodium chloride solution and further boluses as needed.

If meningococcal disease is suspected, intravenous penicillin is given intravenously or intramuscularly immediately and the child is transported to hospital. Intravenous ceftriaxone is given and the intravenous fluid requirement and inotrope support assessed in the intensive care unit.

In children with shock or altered level of consciousness and no source of fever, parenteral ceftriaxone is given and amoxicillin is added if the infant is less than 3 months of age.

Management of fever

The child should be clothed appropriately for the ambient temperature. An antipyretic such as paracetamol or ibuprofen may make the child feel better, but does not prevent febrile convulsions. Cool

Table 27.2 Symptoms and signs of specific diseases.

Diagnosis to be consisdered	Symptoms and signs in conjunction with fever
Meningococcal disease	Non-blanching rash, particularly with one or more of the following: • an ill-looking child • lesions larger than 2 mm in diameter (purpura) • CRT ≥ 3 seconds • neck stiffness
Meningitis*	Neck stiffness Bulging fontanelle Decreased level of consciousness Convulsive status epilepticus
Herpes simplex encephalitis	• Focal neurological signs • Focal seizures • Decreased level of consciousness
Pneumonia	• Tachypnoea, measured as: – 0–5 months – RR > 60 breaths/minute – 6–12 months – RR > 50 breaths/minute – > 12 months – RR > 40 breaths/minute • Crackles in the chest • Nasal flaring • Chest indrawing • Cyanosis • Oxygen saturation ≤ 95%
Urinary tract infection (in children aged older than 3 months)[†]	• Vomiting • Poor feeding • Lethargy • Irritability • Abdominal pain or tenderness • Urinary frequency or dysuria Offensive urine or haematuria
Septic arthritis/osteomyelitis	• Swelling of a limb or joint Not using an extremity Non-using bearing
Kawasaki disease[‡]	Fever lasting longer than 5 days and at least four of the following: bilateral conjunctival injection change in upper respiratory tract mucous membranes (for example, injected pharynx, dry cracked lips or strawberry tongue) change in the peripheral extremities (for example, oedema, erythema or desquamation) polymorphus rash cervical lymphadenopathy

CRT, capillary refill time; RR, respiratory rate.
*Classical signs (neck stiffness, bulging fontanelle, high-pitched cry) are often absent in infants with bacterial meningitis.
[†] Urinary tract infection should be considered in any child aged younger than 3 months with fever (see p. 43).
[‡]In rare cases, incomplete/atypical Kawasaki disease may be diagnosed with fewer features.

baths or tepid sponging are no longer used. Parents are advised to give fluids regularly and to check on their child during the night. Following medical assessment, parents who are looking after their child at home will be given advice on warning signs of deterioration and how to access further advice if needed. In addition, they should be advised to seek further advice if:

• The child has a fit;
• The parent feels that the child is less well than when they previously sought advice;
• They are more worried than when they last sought advice;

• The parent is very distressed or unable to cope with the child's illness; or
• The fever lasts longer than 5 days.

Further reading

National Institute of Clinical Excellence (NICE). *Feverish Illness in Children.* Nice Guideline 47. NICE, 2007.

CHAPTER 28

Behaviour Problems

Bernard Valman

Northwick Park Hospital and Imperial College London, UK

OVERVIEW

- When a child's behaviour worries parents, they seek advice for confirmation of the diagnosis, and advice on management and prognosis.
- The most common behavioural and emotional problems include habitual behaviour, anxiety states, and antisocial behaviour.
- Parents may think that the child has an underlying physical disease.
- Most of these problems resolve spontaneously, but some need professional help.

Habitual behaviour

Many habits are so common that they should be considered as within the normal range. They may provide comfort for stress or anxiety or may be a means of expressing anger, frustration, or boredom. In infancy the most common habits are thumb-sucking, head-banging, and breath-holding attacks. Tics and compulsive behaviour affects mainly schoolchildren. Nail-biting and twirling or pulling hair can affect children of any age. Most habits resolve spontaneously and are not harmful.

Thumb-sucking

A child may suck his thumb when bored, nervous, or in need of comfort. It is most common in children younger than 3 years of age. Some children continue until they are 6–7 years. A rewards system may help the child to stop. About half of all 3-year-olds suck their thumbs.

Nail-biting

About one-third of all children bite their nails. It usually starts during the early years at school and may persist into adulthood. The nail-biting may make the nails unsightly and painful. A young child may give up the habit if distracted when nail-biting occurs and older children may respond to the gift of a nail file, clippers, or scissors.

Head-banging

A child who is frustrated, angry, or bored may bang his head against a hard surface. Such behaviour occurs in a small number of preschool children and usually disappears by the age of 4 years. Although upsetting to the parents, it is seldom harmful to the child. Foam sheeting round the cot or a pillow will soften the impact but otherwise the habit should be ignored. If the symptoms are severe or persistent the advice of behavioural psychologist may be helpful.

Breath-holding attacks

A small number of preschool children habitually hold their breath for periods up to 30 seconds. Rarely, a child becomes unconscious during the episode. An attack may be initiated by pain or frustration, and may be used as a way of manipulating parents. A severe attack may be shortened by distraction – for example, by dropping a spoon – but at other times should be ignored as much as possible. They usually disappear by the age of 4 years.

Tics

Tics are repetitive involuntary movements usually in schoolchildren. The head and face are most often involved and rapid repetitive blinking may occur. Tics are usually the result of stress and in most cases disappear spontaneously within a few months.

If the tic is severe or is accompanied by other disturbances in behaviour the child should be referred to a child psychiatrist or paediatrician.

Compulsions

Schoolchildren often have compulsions, in which they feel the need to perform particular action, such as avoiding cracks in the pavement. Compulsions usually disappear if ignored. If they persist or interfere with normal living – for example, by excessive handwashing – a child psychiatrist should be consulted.

Pulling hair

Children of all ages may twirl or pull their hair from frustration or anxiety. In most children these habits are temporary and require no treatment. Rarely, serious emotional disturbance results in severe hair-pulling and causes bald patches. A child psychiatrist should be consulted for these children.

ABC of One to Seven, 5th edition. Edited by B. Valman. © 2010 Blackwell Publishing, ISBN: 978-1-4051-8105-1.

Anxiety and fears

Anxiety and fears are common in children – for example, when separated from a parent even for a short time. Common causes of anxiety include the dark, loud noises, animals, or strangers. Symptoms of anxiety which may accompany or mimic physical disease include:

- Persistent crying;
- Sleep disturbance;
- Poor appetite;
- Temper tantrums and irritability;
- Recurrent abdominal pain, headaches and limb pains;
- Enuresis and soiling; and
- Tics and compulsions.

Management

If there is a possibility of physical disease it should be investigated and excluded quickly. Possible causes for anxiety should be explored such as being parted from a parent, problems at school or at home, or difficulties with the peer group. If a parent has a fear, the child may adopt it.

By talking with the child it may be possible to discover the cause of anxiety which was unknown to the parent, such as bullying at school. If no cause of anxiety is discovered, the parent should be encouraged to talk with the child at home after an interval. During this period the reason for the anxiety may be found and the child's symptoms may be resolved. If the symptoms are severe and persistent and interfere with daily living, referral to a psychologist or child psychiatrist may be indicated.

Disruptive and antisocial behaviour

All children may have episodes in which they are more disobedient, cheeky, or mischievous. Antisocial behaviour is persistent disobedience and aggressive and disruptive behaviour to a degree that affects a child's development and interferes with the ability of the child and his family to live a normal life.

Symptoms

Disobedience and aggression are found in children with antisocial behaviour at all ages but it takes different forms in the various age groups.

In preschool children:
- Physical attacks on other children or their parents;
- Destruction of objects; or
- Temper tantrums.

In schoolchildren and adolescents:
- Bullying and fighting other children (Figure 28.1);
- Stealing and lying;
- Cruelty to other children or animals;
- Being destructive in class; or
- Truancy and vandalism.

Aggression is usually learnt by example from parents, the peer group, or the media. It is often a symptom of an underlying emotional problem at home or at school. Contributory factors

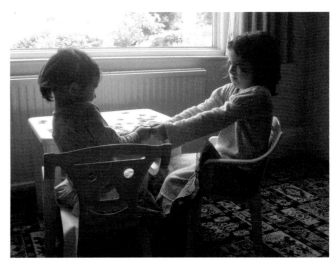

Figure 28.1 Aggression.

may include learning difficulties, attention deficit hyperactivity disorder, or a disability such as deafness.

Management

Parents should talk to their child to try to discover the underlying cause of the symptoms. The parents need to agree a firm, consistent policy which is discussed with the child and which is always implemented. If the symptoms are severe or persistent, referral to a child psychiatrist is indicated. Many children outgrow the behaviour by the age of 15 years. Boys who have severe and prolonged antisocial behaviour are more likely to become antisocial adults.

Chronic fatigue syndrome

This disorder has several names including postviral syndrome. The symptoms may include:

- Severe fatigue that prevents the child from getting out of bed in the morning at the usual time;
- Weakness in the limbs;
- Pain in the head, abdomen, or muscles of the limbs;
- Becoming extremely exhausted after any physical or mental exercise;
- Difficulty in concentrating at school; and
- Reluctance to eat or take part in any social activities.

Management

In a few children the symptoms are preceded by a throat infection or specific viral illness such as infectious mononucleosis. Occasionally, depression causes similar symptoms. Persisting physical disease is excluded by physical examination and blood tests could include erythrocyte sedimentation rate, full blood count, screening test for infectious mononucleosis, liver function tests, throat swab culture, and urine microscopy and culture. The normal results are reassuring to the parents, but should not be repeated.

The child should be encouraged to discuss with the doctor and the parents possible causes of anxiety. A plan for gradual return to full-time school over a fixed period is discussed with and agreed by the child. This plan should ensure steady progress but may take several weeks or months. It should be accompanied by regular monitoring of progress. The problem should be considered resolved when the child is back at school full-time. Failure to improve over a period of 3 weeks or a relapse are indications for referral to a paediatrician or child psychiatrist. The prognosis depends on the length of time that the child has been away from school, and the condition should be suspected and preventive advice given if a child has remained away from school with a trivial illness for over a week or has several prolonged absences.

Further reading

Turk J, Graham P, Verhulst F. *Child and Adolescent Psychiatry: A Developmental Approach*, 4th edn. Oxford University Press, Oxford, 2007.

CHAPTER 29

Children with Special Needs

Daphne Keen

St George's Hospital, London, UK

The parents of a child whose developmental trajectory may be abnormal will want to know what is wrong, the treatment required, the prognosis, and the chances that a future child will have a similar problem. The experience of managing chronic disability will vary from doctor to doctor. Although about 10% of preschool children in a general practice have a chronic disability, most have asthma or behaviour disorders. There are many more children who may be brought by parents worried about developmental variations and learning difficulties, and a general practitioner can help parents considerably if he has an interest in and experience of the normal range of abilities.

Over the past 20 years or so there has been a major change in the morbidity profile of the population of children with disability. There is increasing understanding that some behavioural disorders have neurobiological underpinnings and are driven by underlying developmental disorders. This has been brought about by the increase in recognition of certain conditions, most notably attention deficit hyperactivity disorder (ADHD) and the autism spectrum disorders (ASD) including Asperger's syndrome, which in the past were considered relatively rare conditions. Conversely, there has been a reduction in those described as having uncomplicated learning difficulty. It is very common for the core problems of ADHD and ASD to present together with other developmental impairments and/or mental health problems. Both conditions are associated with higher risk of impaired motor skills (motor clumsiness), disruptive behaviours, sleep disorders, and chronic tic or Tourette's disorder. Associated anxiety and mood disorders may give added complexity to presentation, assessment, and management of these conditions.

A general practitioner is likely to see one new case of Down's syndrome every 10 years. A district paediatric unit may have about 100 patients with cerebral palsy and 250 with ADHD under their care, and assess 30–40 new cases of ASD per year (Table 29.1).

About 1 in 1000 children has severe hearing loss and this is managed mainly at special centres, but many children in every general practice have fluctuating or persistent hearing loss resulting from secretory otitis media. Severe visual defects are often associated with other abnormalities, but defects in visual acuity, which could

Table 29.1 Prevalence of children with special needs.

Disorder	Rate per 1000 children
Learning problem	30
Autism spectrum disorders	10
Attention deficit hyperactivity disorder	50
Cerebral palsy	3
Epilepsy	6
Asthma	100
Blindness	0.25
Refractive error	50
Hearing defects	
Mild, usually caused by glue ear	50
Moderate (need hearing aid)	2
Severely deaf	1

be corrected by refraction, often pass undetected for long periods. Although a family doctor may have only two children with epilepsy in the practice, a district's epilepsy service will be following up well over 100 in its outpatient clinics.

Chronic disabilities affecting the central nervous system or special senses are rare in general practice. They are not simply medical problems and their adequate assessment needs the help of several disciplines, including the social and educational services. Most of these children are referred to their local district developmental paediatrician and their management illustrates important aspects of child care.

Identifying a developmental disorder

There is an enormous variation as to when different types of developmental disorders are typically first identified. Some conditions may be diagnosed prenatally or are evident soon after birth, for example, Down's and other syndromes or myelomeningocele. Others, such as Asperger's syndrome, can – despite the child having obvious difficulties – go unrecognized in childhood and are only picked up when the young adult presents to an astute professional.

A doctor may discover that the child has developmental delay at a routine assessment clinic, during a consultation for an acute illness,

ABC of One to Seven, 5th edition. Edited by B. Valman. © 2010 Blackwell Publishing, ISBN: 978-1-4051-8105-1.

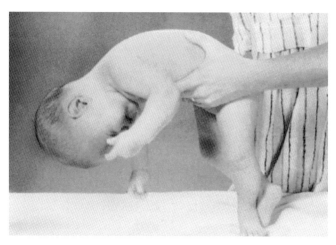

Figure 29.1 Developmental delay with hypotonia.

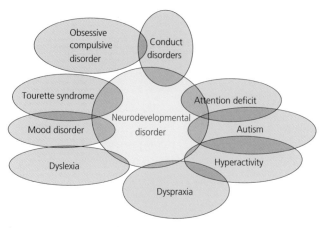

Figure 29.2 The overlap of developmental disorders.

or while following up a child of low birth weight (Figure 29.1). Mothers may raise questions with their health visitors when they visit the home or at the clinic, and health visitors play an important part in encouraging mothers to report their fears and in arranging referrals. A neighbour, relative, or friend may notice that an infant is not performing like her own child of that age and may point it out to the parents. Parents may compare one child with a sibling or, not uncommonly, have read books and accessed information on the Internet on child development. Parents are usually correct in their suspicions. Unfortunately, it is still not uncommon for parents to be incorrectly reassured by health professionals that all is well or that the child will 'grow out of' the problem. Failure to recognize a serious developmental problem may lay the foundations for later distrust of medical advice.

If the parent suspects that their child is developing and behaving unusually, a prompt referral should be made to a consultant paediatrician specializing in child development or disability.

Assessment process

Initial consultation

The configuration of child development services varies enormously both by district and the nature of the suspected problem. This sometimes causes primary care staff difficulty in negotiating referral pathways. The situation for conditions such as suspected cerebral palsy or sensory impairment is usually clear but that for the neurodevelopmental disorders such as ADHD and ASD can vary considerably. Increasingly, paediatric services are taking a leading role in assessment and management of ADHD, ASD, and related conditions but, depending on local skills and expertise, the Child and Adolescent Mental Health (CAMHS) team may have responsibility, and sometimes this is shared between services.

An expert paediatric assessment through detailed history and examination is essential for all children with developmental concerns. This is because there is a high likelihood of other associated medical and developmental conditions being identified. Patients are referred to consultant paediatricians by general practitioners, community doctors, therapists, and health visitors as well as by nursery and educational professionals.

For those with suspected physical disability, the family may be seen for initial assessment by the consultant alone or jointly with one or more members of the multidisciplinary team (MDT), such as speech and language therapists, occupational therapists, or physiotherapists. Those with suspected language and communication disorders may be seen by the consultant alone or jointly with a speech and language therapist or clinical psychologist.

The initial history and examination may lead to an immediate firm diagnosis but in other situations there may be uncertainty as to whether there is deviation from the normal range or whether a more complex and multifaceted condition is present (Figure 29.2). Significant past or current psychosocial adversity cause additional complexity and a longer term programme of assessment and observation will be necessary. At this stage, either a definitive or provisional diagnosis can be given and investigations may be indicated: biochemical, genetic, neurophysiological, and imaging studies. Alternatively, further investigation may be delayed until the nature of the problem becomes clearer.

These results and further assessments will be discussed with the parents at the next visit with an agreed programme of management.

Assessment process

The core MDT will decide who should see the child to continue the assessment. An audiological examination is essential for all children with developmental delays and most of those with neurological disabilities will need to be seen by an ophthalmologist and orthoptist. The MDT will involve other colleagues as necessary such as a clinical or educational psychologist, specialist social worker, and clinical nurse specialist as well as consultant colleagues in related disciplines such as neurology, orthopaedics, genetics, or psychiatry of learning disability.

Therapists may assess over a single period of time or take the opportunity to assess the child in different settings such as during a meal and at play as well as by formal tests. Assessment for suspected ASD or ADHD will often involve observation of how a child learns and relates to their peer group in a nursery or classroom setting and will usually involve collection of information from a variety of observers and using recognized interview schedules and assessment tools.

Management and interventions

Generally, the whole MDT will meet to agree on the diagnosis and management plan before meeting with the family again. Ideally, a 'key worker' will be selected to coordinate interventions, liaise with key agencies, avoid duplicating treatment, and give the parents a person to telephone in a crisis.

Many centres compile a written report for parents, shared with professionals, detailing the findings of assessment and the management plan. The team then sits down with the parents to discuss the diagnosis, management, and prognosis. Other important professionals may be invited to attend – for example, the family's health visitor may provide the team with an insight into family dynamics and provide support at subsequent home visits. Nursery and teaching staff can bring helpful information about the child's life at school and then help in implementing intervention plans. The parents should be given an ample opportunity to discuss their worries and should be encouraged to write down important things they want to discuss which saves forgetting important points. Some parents may wish to discuss these points with the consultant alone as they may be intimidated by the large team.

Therapists, by seeing patients in their own homes, nurseries, and schools are well placed to advise on practical management. Whereas a specific course of one-to-one hospital or centre-based therapy will always have an important role, whether for developing motor skills or those of language and communication, increasingly therapists focus on teaching and supporting parents/carers, nursery and teaching staff in how to consolidate interventions and help the child on a day-to-day basis. For example, an occupational therapy programme to develop skills in dressing can be embedded into a PE class routine and a social skills group working on conversational turn-taking may help a child with autism to form social relationships with peers. Taking children out of school for treatment has the disadvantage of accentuating the stigma of being different and can be disruptive to school life.

Such intervention programmes may be incorporated into special needs provision through an Individual Education Plan (IEP) and may proceed to formal status through a Statement of Special Educational Need (see below). Details of the 1993 Education Act are given on page 130.

Many families with children with disability will benefit from social work support at some stage and medical social workers work closely with disability services. Many districts provide respite care for children with severe disabilities to enable their carers to recover from a crisis or take a short holiday. Provision is also made for specialist play schemes in school holidays.

Children with significant disability, whether physical, intellectual, or, in some cases, behavioural, are entitled to receive a Disability Living Allowance. To support an application, a medical statement is requested either from the consultant or by the general practitioner if he knows the child well. The services provided by the regional genetics service should be discussed with all parents even if they are not contemplating a new pregnancy in the near future.

Parental reactions

Initially, young parents or parents of firstborn children may have difficulty in persuading a doctor that the child is developing abnormally. This may delay the diagnosis or cause frustration and considerable subsequent hostility to all medical advisers. Parents must be told the truth about their child or, if uncertain, the concerns professionals hold, and all aspects of the prognosis should be discussed honestly. In common with other situations when people receive bad news, individual reactions can be unpredictable and diverse. Many parents are shocked when the diagnosis is discussed and can feel detached or overwhelmed. The reality of the symptoms may be denied, the doctor's competence questioned, and the parents may search for an alternative opinion.

It is preferable that both parents be present when the diagnosis is explained so that they can support each other, or perhaps a close family member or friend. A follow-up meeting might be necessary shortly afterwards to go over areas of difficulty or answer new questions.

Parents may become increasingly dispirited and mourn for the 'normal' child they have lost (Figure 29.3). They may blame themselves for the child's problems and deep anxiety – for example, about events during pregnancy – may continue to cause anguish over the years. Some parents deny the diagnosis for some time and others may continue to do so for several years, perhaps coming back to ask for clarification repeatedly. Some seem unable to understand anything but the simplest information.

Both parents may develop protracted symptoms of grief with typical symptoms of depression or preoccupation with the child. Primary care staff should be alert to the negative effects of grief reactions on relationships within the family: between parents, between parent and the affected child, between parents and siblings. These symptoms can lead to hostility towards the professionals caring for the child. Siblings may develop behaviour problems because their parents seem to be remote and uncaring. Health visitors may be able to help the parents through the process because they are already familiar to the parents and so may avoid the hostility that the parents may feel towards those who have diagnosed the disability.

Not all parents, however, will experience distressing reactions to their child's problem. Many have a philosophical or religious outlook that is accepting of what others may consider adversity.

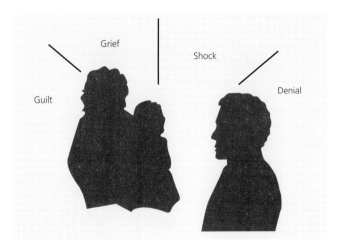

Figure 29.3 Parental reactions.

Some may feel relieved that the diagnosis has confirmed their suspicions and, having already passed through a bereavement reaction, feel positive that an effective treatment plan can begin soon.

Early and appropriate treatment also helps parents to understand how to help their child and can give a sense of empowerment. Supporting parents can indirectly be beneficial to the child, for example, the Early Bird parent programme developed by the National Autistic Society and run by many services.

Training junior staff in the management of these children is difficult. Most trainees can see a child over only a year, and families usually need support for much longer. Confidence in the doctor and ability to discuss problems with him is attained only after a long period and is not easily transferred.

Voluntary sector and parents' groups

Increasingly important is the role of the voluntary sector in parental support. These may be specialist organizations, for example, providing respite care or condition-specific parent advice services, or generic family support organizations offering services to all families with children who have special needs. Most associations also raise money for research but all enable parents of children with similar problems to make best use of local resources and discuss mutual problems.

Many parents find the help available from parent support organizations extremely important (and often more helpful than professionals) in providing contact with other parents in a similar situation who understand their experiences. Details of such organizations are held by child development teams and associated medical social workers and clinical nurse specialists.

Education

The Children Act 1989 has introduced the concept of children in need and the disability register, and details are found on page 141.

Children identified as having likely special educational needs are formally notified by paediatricians or child development teams to the special needs department of the local education authority. Depending on the severity of need, progression to a statutory assessment of special educational need may be made. Many children can be supported satisfactorily without this provision through the special needs resources allocated to mainstream schools, but all those in special schools or units are likely to have a Statement. Every school will have a special needs coordinator (SENCO) who will be the key person to lead educational support and arrange for the educational psychologist to assess support needs.

Local education authorities have to provide some form of education provision for children with special needs from the age of 2 years and to provide the necessary transport if needed. Facilities for preschool children with special needs, however, can vary considerably from district to district. For many young infants with significant disability, the Portage home intervention programme will be offered early on. This teaches mothers how to develop skills of the child by graded exercises to reach defined objectives.

In some areas, specialist day centres, nurseries, or playgroups are available for children from around 2 years of age. Some education authorities provide specialist nursery places within special schools for children with physical disability, intellectual disability, or autism. In such specialist settings there is a high staff to child ratio, and therapy provision (occupational, speech and language therapists or physiotherapist) incorporated into the nursery activities. However, most children with special needs will go to mainstream primary schools and recent reorganization of special education reflects current parental preference for mainstream education, at least for the primary stage.

Further reading

Voluntary sector

Contact a Family: for families with disabled children offering information on specific conditions and rare disorders. www.cafamily.org.uk

National Attention Deficit Disorder Information and Support Service (ADDISS): information and resources about ADHD for parents, patients, teachers, and health professionals. www.addiss.co.uk

National Autistic Society. www.nas.org.uk/

CHAPTER 30

School Failure

Ruth Levere

Child and Adolescent Mental Health Services, Harrow, UK

OVERVIEW

- School failure is usually the result of a complex interaction of factors.
- Child factors include physical, sensory, intellectual, specific learning, neurodevelopmental, and emotional difficulties.
- Family factors include lack of support for learning and unrealistic expectations.
- School factors include the assessment regime, bullying, and a wide range of needs in the class.
- Doctors need to decide which children require further assessment and refer accordingly.

Parents must by law ensure that their children are educated between the ages of 5 and 16 and the local authority has a duty to provide appropriate schools and teachers. There are also independent schools which include fee-paying establishments and, more recently, academies. Furthermore, increasing numbers of children are home-educated, some having previously experienced school failure. All maintained schools have to teach the National Curriculum and there are a series of educational assessments, known as SATs (Standard Assessment Tests), to assess children's attainments in literacy, numeracy, and science.

Child and parental attitudes to school are variable but most children start school with positive anticipation and support from parents. Unfortunately, often not long into their school experience, some children experience failure which leads to a negative attitude, unhappiness, and sometimes refusal to attend.

When parents are told initially that their child is experiencing problems at school they may have a good idea of what the relevant issues are – for example, recent parental separation – or they may attribute the problem to the child or the school. It is usual for schools to try to address school failure through their own resources in the first instance, such as extra teaching or referral to a learning mentor or school counsellor. If this is not successful the school or parents may decide to involve external support such as the educational psychology service. In some cases, either because there are indications of a medical issue such as attention deficit hyperactivity disorder

(ADHD) or in order to bypass the educational route because of the length of the waiting list, parents may be asked to discuss the problem with their general practitioner. GPs would normally refer to the local Child and Adolescent Mental Health Service (CAMHS) but unless there is an indication of a mental health problem as opposed to an educational one, such as dyslexia, the referral will be rejected. Although such services may employ professionals such as child clinical psychologists who can assess learning problems they are only resourced to do this within the context of a mental health assessment.

There are many different reasons for children failing in school and broadly they can be divided into intrinsic or child-related factors and extrinsic, environmental causes. Intrinsic causes include intellectual disability, specific learning difficulties, ADHD and autism spectrum disorder (ASD). Extrinsic causes relate to either home issues, such as parental separation, or the school setting (e.g. poor teaching). However, in most cases there is not a single cause of school failure but rather it is the result of a complex interaction of child, family, social, and school factors.

Child factors

Absence from school

Teachers aim to help children acquire basic skills in a logical, progressive sequence. A child who is often absent from school may have great difficulty filling in the gaps (Box 30.1). Frequent short absences may prove more damaging educationally than a prolonged absence because teachers may not realize the child is missing so much schooling. It is important to establish how much school a child is missing and why. The child may be physically unwell or could have psychosomatic symptoms caused by anxiety.

Physical and sensory difficulties

Although children may have their hearing and vision checked during the preschool years it is still possible to miss, for example, a fluctuating conductive hearing loss. Concerned parents are good observers of their children and it is worth questioning them about their views of their child's hearing and vision. Some children have gross and/or fine motor coordination difficulties which impact on their learning and require assessment by a paediatric occupational therapist.

ABC of One to Seven, 5th edition. Edited by B. Valman. © 2010 Blackwell Publishing, ISBN: 978-1-4051-8105-1.

Box 30.1 **Child factors**

- School absence
- Physical and sensory difficulties
- Intellectual difficulties
- Specific learning difficulties
- Neurodevelopmental problems
- Emotional difficulties
- Mental health problems

Intellectual difficulties

Teachers do not expect all children to learn at the same pace but some children are much slower than those at the slow end of a wide normal range. Although children whose preschool development has been abnormally slow would usually have been identified by school age, the policy of integrating children with special needs in mainstream education results in some children with a moderate learning disability being placed initially in school with little support. This sometimes happens when a specific delay, usually in language development, has been identified but it has not been recognized that the child has global intellectual difficulties.

Specific learning difficulties

Although not unintelligent some children have great difficulty in mastering the basic skills of literacy and numeracy, despite regular teaching. There is controversy over the use of the term 'dyslexia' to describe a specific reading difficulty, because of the problems of both definition and causation. Some severely delayed readers have spatial and sequencing difficulties whereas others find it hard to perceive and analyse sounds.

It is being increasingly recognized that children can have other specific difficulties that impact on their learning. Some children have short or long-term memory problems. Others who fail to progress at school may have problems with executive functioning as exemplified by poor planning or organizational skills. However, these difficulties are usually only identified if a child has a neuropsychological assessment, usually for a reason other than poor progress at school.

Neurodevelopmental problems

Children with ADHD and ASD often have associated learning problems. Both conditions can coexist with any level of intellectual ability and are associated with specific learning difficulties.

The attention problems, overactivity and impulsiveness which characterize ADHD can result in the child being unable to access the teaching in a busy classroom (Figure 30.1). Children with ADHD usually have a combination of symptoms that place them in one of three subtypes: ADHD mainly inattentive; ADHD mainly hyperactive–impulsive; and ADHD combined type. Parents sometimes find it hard to understand that their child can receive a diagnosis of ADHD when they do not show major symptoms of hyperactivity.

Children with ASD may also have attention problems but in addition may show a number of behaviours such as poor motivation, social skills difficulties, and restricted interests which result in them not achieving academically.

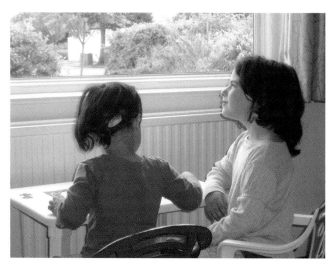

Figure 30.1 Attention problems.

Where the doctor suspects that a child may be showing signs of ADHD or ASD he should refer to the local child development or CAMHS service for a comprehensive assessment. A child clinical psychologist working as a team member has a role in the assessment and management of the behaviour difficulties which are often shown by children with ADHD and ASD in both school and home.

Emotional difficulties

A child who is failing at school will almost always have accompanying emotional distress which may then exacerbate the learning difficulties. However, for many children, emotional distress may be the outcome of their personal and social environment. Children who are experiencing domestic violence or any form of abuse, parental separation, or parental physical or mental illness are likely to be distressed and may express this in behaviour problems in school. Unfortunately, some of these circumstances, notably family breakdown, are so common and children's distress so understandable that referral to CAMHS is not appropriate. Parents have to be told that the problem is not located in the child but that it is the parents' responsibility to work out their own problems in a way that minimizes the harm done to their children.

Mental health problems

Rarely, a young child will have a diagnosable mental health problem such as anxiety, depression, or obsessive compulsive disorder which will result in a child not being able to concentrate on learning. If any of these conditions are suspected referral should be made to CAMHS so that a full assessment can take place and suggestions made as to how the child can be helped in the school setting.

Family factors

The impact parents have on the academic success of their children is immeasurable. In order to succeed most children need parents/carers who are involved, value learning, and maintain a good relationship with the school. However, some parents can be over-involved and have unrealistic expectations for their child which

Box 30.2 **Family factors**

- Lack of support for learning
- Unrealistic expectations
- Poor relationship with school

Box 30.3 **School factors**

- Stressed teachers
- Wide range of needs in class
- Bullying
- SATs and other assessments

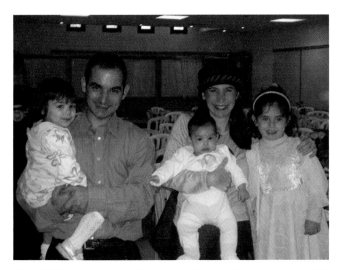

Figure 30.2 Eighty per cent of academic achievement is related to parental support.

result in a sense of failure, poor self-esteem, and disengagement with education (Box 30.2).

Modern lifestyles involving either a single working parent or two working parents often result in children spending long days in school. Where children attend a school breakfast club they may be tired before learning in the classroom begins. At home parents often do not have time to support their child in reading and sometimes prefer to spend what time they do have in doing things they perceive as fun rather than work.

Research has shown that the effect of parents and what they do at home to support learning can account for 80% of a child's academic success (Figure 30.2). This compares with schools being directly responsible for around 20% of factors leading to academic attainment. Thus, the importance of family factors cannot be underestimated.

School factors

There are poor teachers but more frequently there are good or adequate teachers working under very stressful conditions who are expected to teach children who live chaotic lives outside school (Box 30.3). Furthermore, in many classes the range of ability levels, languages spoken, and parental attitudes can be very wide and not all children have the resilience to learn in such settings. Bullying is also a major issue in some schools leading to emotional distress and school failure. Finally, the assessment regime of regular SATs and other tests is thought by some to put young children under unnecessary stress.

Summary

In summary, there are multiple causes of school failure: some primarily educational, others primarily social, and some related to medical conditions. There are many sources of and layers of support for children and it is the role of the GP to identify which children require a paediatric or CAMHS assessment and advise parents of children who do not need such an assessment where they can go for appropriate support.

Further reading

ADHD information: www.addiss.co.uk

ASD information: www.autism.org.uk

Dyslexia information: www.bda-dyslexia.org.uk

Turk J, Graham P, Verhulst F. *Child and Adolescent Psychiatry: A Developmental Approach*, 4th edn. Oxford University Press, Oxford, 2007. (especially Chapter 3, Neurodevelopment and neuropsychiatric disorders)

CHAPTER 31

Minor Orthopaedic Problems

John Fixsen

Great Ormond Street Children's Hospital, London, UK

OVERVIEW

- Minor orthopaedic problems such as in-toeing, bow legs, knock knees, and flat feet cause anxiety both to parents and doctors (Box 31.1).
- In-toeing is nearly always caused by one of three conditions: metatarsus varus, which affects the foot; medial tibial torsion, which affects the lower leg; and persistent femoral anteversion, which affects the whole leg.
- In managing all these minor orthopaedic anomalies the whole child must be examined to ensure that the orthopaedic problem is not part of a more serious generalized disorder.

Box 31.1 Minor orthopaedic problems

- In-toeing
- Bow legs
- Knock knees
- Flat feet

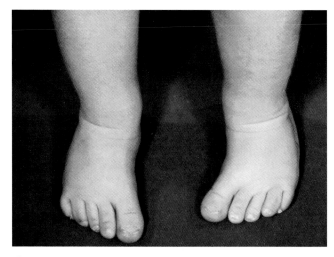

Figure 31.1 Metatarsus varus.

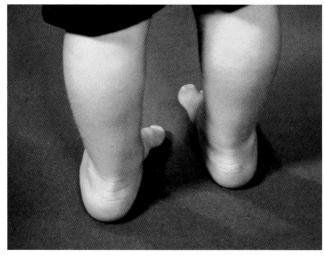

Figure 31.2 Metatarsus varus.

Metatarsus varus or adductus

Metatarsus varus or adductus, hookfoot, or skewfoot, is very common. It may be noticed at or soon after birth but is most obvious and causes most anxiety when the child starts to walk. At this stage the child falls frequently. Parents often ascribe the falls to the pronounced in-toeing rather than to the complex problem of learning bipedal gait. Metatarsus varus can be distinguished from talipes equino varus as only the forefoot is abnormal (Figures 31.1 and 31.2). The heel is in line with the leg (Figure 31.3) and the foot can be flexed to 90° or more.

Ninety per cent of all cases of metatarsus varus correct spontaneously without treatment by the age of 3–4 years. Most of the remaining children will have no complaints about their feet; a few will show persistent deformity that will require treatment with plasters and occasionally surgery. When advising parents to wait for natural resolution in the face of obvious deformity it is important to explain three things: first, the natural history and high spontaneous recovery rate; secondly, the time recovery is likely to take; and thirdly, that if their child is the 'odd man out' who does not correct then adequate and full correction is possible and has not been jeopardized by waiting.

Medial tibial torsion

Medial tibial torsion is nearly always associated with outward curving of the tibia, which is an exaggeration of the normal or

---

ABC of One to Seven, 5th edition. Edited by B. Valman. © 2010 Blackwell Publishing, ISBN: 978-1-4051-8105-1.

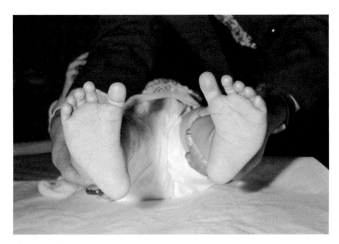

Figure 31.3 Metatarsus varus.

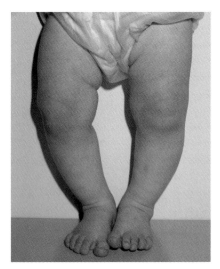

Figure 31.4 Physiological bowing.

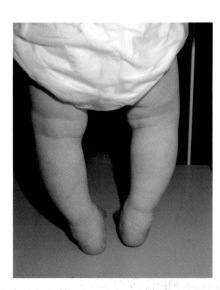

Figure 31.5 Physiological bowing.

physiological bowing of the tibia (Figure 31.4 and 31.5). In medial tibial torsion when the knee is pointing forwards the foot is medially rotated 20–30° whereas in the adult the foot is normally rotated outwards 0–25°. Both the medial torsion and the bowing should correct spontaneously by the age of 3–4 years provided that they are not associated with any other abnormality. No special shoes or splints are necessary. Beware of pronounced unilateral bowing, which suggests an epiphyseal abnormality. Anterior bowing by contrast is nearly always important and requires investigation.

Tibia vara and rickets

Tibia vara (Blount's disease), caused by epiphyseal growth abnormality, should be considered, particularly in West Indian and West African children, if the bowing is very pronounced and the angulation immediately below the knee (Figure 31.6).

Dietary rickets should also be considered, particularly among immigrant children with pronounced bowing of the tibiae (Figure 31.7). Swelling round the knees, wrists, and ankles, craniotabes, Harrison's sulcus, and a 'rachitic rosary' should also be looked for.

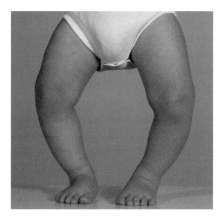

Figure 31.6 Tibia vara.

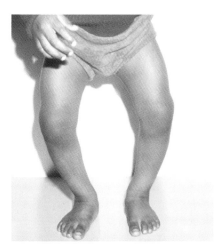

Figure 31.7 Rickets.

Persistent femoral anteversion and retroversion

In persistent femoral anteversion the whole leg turns in from the hip. The patellae look towards each other – so-called squinting patellae. The child characteristically sits between the legs (Figure 31.8). To demonstrate the femoral neck anteversion the child should be examined prone with the hips extended and the knees flexed. Internal rotation of the hip is greater than external rotation and can easily be seen and measured. In 80% of these children the anteversion will correct by the age of 8 years. It is doubtful whether any form of special shoe or splint can influence the condition. If there is severe, persistent, functional and cosmetic deformity after the age of 8 femoral osteotomy is occasionally indicated.

Femoral retroversion (out-toeing) is the opposite condition. The child lies or stands with the legs externally rotated 90° (Figure 31.9). There is often no internal rotation in extension at the hip. This condition corrects within a year of the child starting to walk. It is important to check the extent of abduction in flexion of the hips carefully as congenital dislocation of the hip can also cause external rotation.

Knock knees

Seventy five per cent of children aged 2–4½ years have some degree of intermalleolar separation; up to 9 cm measured with the child lying down is acceptable (Figure 31.10). There is no evidence that shoe modification, splints, or exercises affect this condition. It is important to look for pronounced asymmetry, short stature, and other skeletal abnormalities which may indicate a more serious problem. If the intermalleolar distance is more than 9 cm an anteroposterior radiograph of both legs on the same film is probably the most useful radiological investigation as it will not only show the knee deformity but also the hip and ankle joints and the whole of the long bones of the legs on one film. If the condition does not correct spontaneously medial epiphyseal stapling at 10–11 years or corrective osteotomy at maturity is the treatment of choice.

Flat feet

There are two forms of flat feet: the first are pain free and have normal mobility and normal muscle power; the second are painful and stiff, or hypermobile, and show abnormal muscle power – that is, they are weak or spastic (Figure 31.11). The simplest method of testing is to ask the patient to stand on tiptoe. If the arches are restored by this simple test then the feet are almost certainly normal.

It is important to remember that the normal foot is flat when the child starts to stand. The medial arch does not develop until the second or third year of life. Most children with flat feet will fall

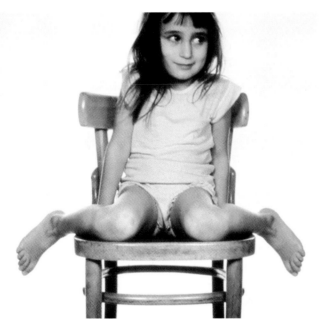

Figure 31.8 Femoral anteversion.

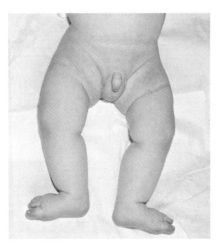

Figure 31.9 Femoral retroversion.

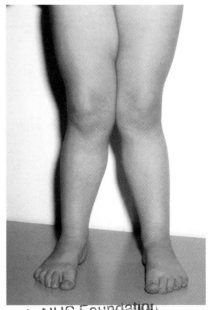

Figure 31.10 Knock knee.

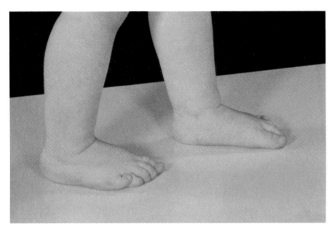

Figure 31.11 Flat feet.

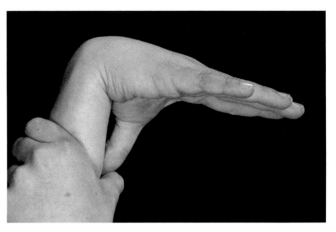

Figure 31.12 Joint laxity.

into the first group. These characteristics are commonly familial or racial. Treatment with insoles, shoe modification, or exercises is unlikely to make any difference to the shape of the feet. Shoe wear can be a problem and insoles or medial stiffening may help. Surgery is rarely indicated. The second group is important as there is either a local bony or inflammatory problem in the foot that needs diagnosis and treatment or the flat foot is part of a more generalized condition such as severe generalized joint laxity, cerebral palsy, peroneal spastic flat foot, or Down's syndrome.

Joint laxity

Joint laxity should always be considered in children with a clumsy or awkward gait. The presence of three or more of the following is evidence of definite joint laxity: in the arm, hyperextension of the wrist and metacarpophalangeal joints, the thumb, or the elbow; in the leg, hyperextension of the knee or ankle (Figure 31.12). Laxity is often familial or racial. It may be part of a generalized disorder such as osteogenesis imperfecta, Ehlers–Danlos syndrome, or Marfan's syndrome.

When counselling parents about minor orthopaedic problems it is important to examine the patient fully, to explain the natural history of the condition, and to check carefully for more serious disorders.

Further reading

Hutson JM, O'Brien M, Beaseley SW, eds. *Jones' Clinical Paediatric Surgery: Diagnosis and Management*, 6th edn. Wiley-Blackwell, Oxford, 2008.

CHAPTER 32

Limp

John Fixsen

Great Ormond Street Children's Hospital, London, UK

Children with a limp may have a minor injury which will recover spontaneously in a few hours or a condition that may affect them for life if treatment is delayed. A diagnosis must be made or, if this is not possible, the children should be observed if necessary in hospital until they have fully recovered. A full history and careful examination of the whole child is essential. A radiograph of the affected area is taken, but pain in the thigh and knee referred from the hip can lead to the wrong area being examined. Parents' observations may sometimes sound odd but should not be dismissed. Abnormal physical signs are usually present in any child with a limp that has a serious cause. Limp may be caused by pain, leg inequality, neuromuscular dysfunction, or, rarely, psychological disturbance. These groups often overlap. Ultrasound is the best method of detecting a joint effusion, especially in the hip.

Pain

The most common cause of limp is pain. Injury may produce muscle strain or fractures but non-accidental injury or a foreign body should always be considered. Any pain that does not settle within a few days or recurs should be investigated. Perthes' disease, slipped upper femoral epiphysis (Figure 32.1), and benign tumours such as osteoid osteoma often produce intermittent pain, which can easily be dismissed as a recurrent muscle strain.

Irritable hip

Irritable hip (transient synovitis, observation hip, coxalgia fugax) is a common condition of unknown cause. The child suddenly starts limping and there is spasm of the hip muscles but no other abnormal signs. The child may have a mild fever and raised erythrocyte sedimentation rate. Transient synovitis usually settles with a short period of bed rest. Traction is helpful to relieve muscle spasm and pain. Most children have no further problems, but a few may have recurrent attacks and subsequently develop changes of Perthes' disease or juvenile arthritis. It is important to eliminate more serious conditions such as septic arthritis or osteomyelitis, Perthes' disease, juvenile chronic arthritis, slipped upper femoral epiphysis (which

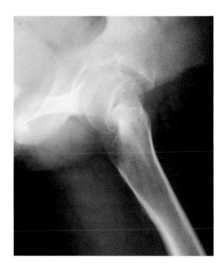

Figure 32.1 Slipped upper femoral epiphysis.

is outside the age group of this book), tuberculosis and, rarely, tumours and leukaemia.

Septic arthritis

The child with septic arthritis is usually seriously ill but beware of the child with immunodeficiency, immunosuppression, or who has been given a short course of antibiotics that mask the signs and symptoms. Perthes' disease and slipped upper femoral epiphysis should be seen on a radiograph. It is important to take a frog lateral view as well as an anteroposterior view of the hips to diagnose and evaluate these two conditions. Juvenile chronic arthritis and tuberculosis are likely to have a longer time course and also show radiographic changes.

Perthes' disease

Treatment for Perthes' disease is confusing both to the general practitioner and the orthopaedic surgeon. There is evidence that suggests that Perthes' disease is caused by temporary ischaemia of the femoral head. Treatment cannot prevent the disease but is aimed at improving the outcome. Many patients need no treatment after the acute episode of pain and spasm. Regular radiographic monitoring of the hip is necessary to ensure that the femoral head remains within the acetabulum (Figure 32.2). If the femoral head

ABC of One to Seven, 5th edition. Edited by B. Valman. © 2010 Blackwell Publishing, ISBN: 978-1-4051-8105-1.

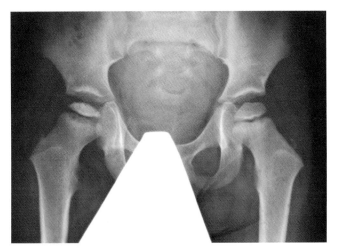

Figure 32.2 Perthes' disease.

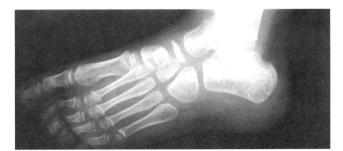

Figure 32.3 Osteochondrosis.

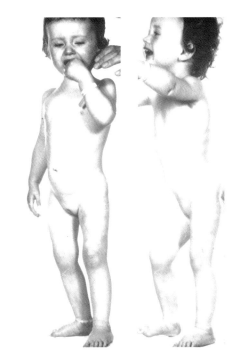

Figure 32.4 Congenital dislocation of the hip.

begins to move out of the acetabulum abduction splints, plasters, or surgery may be needed to achieve containment of the head.

Osteochondroses

Osteochondritis of the tarsal navicular may cause pain over the medial arch of the foot. A radiograph will confirm the diagnosis (Figure 32.3). Most cases settle with reduction of activity. Sometimes a short period in plaster below the knee is necessary. Osteochondritis affecting the heel or the tibial tubercle and osteochondritis dissecans of the knee rarely occur in this age group.

Other causes of pain

Verrucas, foreign bodies, and minor fractures may also cause pain in the foot. Persistent swelling, particularly around the ankle, suggests juvenile chronic arthritis, which commonly presents in the foot in children.

In this age group pain around the knee is rare although it becomes increasingly common in early adolescence. Causes of pain in the knee include bone and joint sepsis, chronic inflammatory conditions, and mechanical derangement such as a discoid meniscus.

Leg inequality

A short leg must be distinguished from apparent shortening resulting from pelvic obliquity, scoliosis, or joint deformity. Congenital

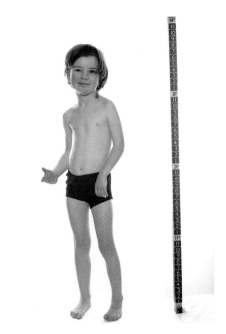

Figure 32.5 Cerebral palsy.

defects such as short femur or tibia are usually obvious. Despite early screening programmes, congenital dislocation of the hip must always be considered. Typically, the leg is short and externally rotated, and abduction in flexion is limited (Figure 32.4). The child usually walks with the leg straight on the dislocated side and the knee flexed on the normal side. The doctor may consider that the flexed knee is abnormal and fail to recognize that the opposite hip is abnormal. Hemiplegic cerebral palsy, spinal dysraphism, and

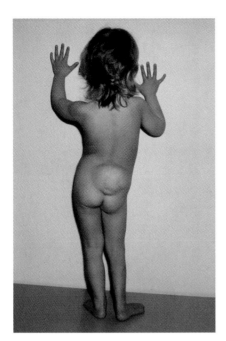

Figure 32.6 Spinal tumour.

poliomyelitis cause poor growth of the affected leg and can be detected by a neurological examination. The whole spine should be examined for the warning signs of dysraphism: a naevus, hairy patch, pit, or lipoma. Epiphyseal injury from trauma or sepsis can cause shortening and deformity.

Neuromuscular and emotional disorders

Complex disturbances of gait, such as incoordination or weakness resulting from cerebral palsy (Figure 32.5), muscular dystrophy, or spinal or cerebral tumour (Figure 32.6) may be described by the parents as a limp. A careful history and examination will usually suggest the diagnosis.

If a limp has an emotional origin diagnosis may be difficult. Usually, the pattern of gait is bizarre and the physical signs inconsistent. It is essential to eliminate any possible organic cause. Often it is necessary to admit the patient to hospital for a few days' observation. A bone scan is a most useful investigation, both to eliminate the possibility of abnormality in the bone that has not been detected by radiographs and to show up hot or cold areas before radiographic changes are present.

Further reading

Hutson JM, O'Brien M, Beaseley SW, eds. *Jones' Clinical Paediatric Surgery: Diagnosis and Management*, 6th edn. Wiley-Blackwell, Oxford, 2008.

CHAPTER 33

Services for Children: Primary Care

Ed Peile

University of Warwick, Coventry, UK

> **OVERVIEW**
>
> - Primary care services for children are in a state of flux in the light of recent policy documents.
> - More acute care for children and more care for continuing illness in children are happening outside of hospital, as paediatric admissions are becoming rarer and shorter.
> - However services are delivered, general practice teams will continue to have a key role.
> - The key to good care for children is effective collaboration between all the professionals involved, with attention to training needs.

Primary care services for children are provided in various service configurations by general practice teams and by paediatric and community child health staff. General practitioners (GPs) offer care for the whole family in both preventive and curative medicine, supported by specialists in the community or hospital.

About 25% of GP workload concerns children, and the Royal College of General Practitioners (RCGP) curriculum for care of children and young people emphasizes the problem-solving skills that help GPs to offer safe and effective care, recognizing that, because children are dependent and developing, their needs are different from those of patients in other age groups. The average GP cares for about 500 children. In the first year of life they will consult about four or five times on average and less than twice a year is the average from 1 to 15 years. Parents, carers, and children need unfettered access to medical care, an increasing proportion of which is provided by telephone, and less by home visits, but still 84% of general practice consultations happen in the GP surgery. In urban areas an increasing proportion of urgent care for children is provided in paediatric assessment units at hospital locations.

In general practices, doctors undertake 62% of all consultations, focusing on acute and chronic illness. Nurses, including health visitors, undertake 34% of general practice consultations, and provide, through appropriate team care, various preventive services such as child health surveillance and asthma clinics. Children with special needs require close collaboration between primary and secondary care teams for optimal care. However skilled, GPs remain generalists and a key skill is effective team-working with other members of the primary health care team (PHCT) and with other professionals and teams.

As hospital services for children are reconfigured, so there is increased emphasis on providing integrated children's health care in the community.

General practice organization

The main aim of the practice should be to make consultation accessible and effective. The appointment system should be flexible enough to accommodate an anxious parent with a sick child, offering appointment possibilities to suit the working parent. There should be a room to isolate children with unidentified rashes and known infectious diseases.

The waiting area should have safe, clean toys and reading matter appropriate to a range of ages. Attention paid to safety issues such as radiator covers and safety plugs should be explicit in order to set a good example for parents. The waiting room presents useful opportunities for health information and health promotion. Attractive noticeboards with regularly updated information may also include community information about toddler groups and even small ads for outgrown children's equipment, leading parents and carers to explore leaflets about child health issues such as accident prevention, immunization, and common illnesses. Such information is sometimes supplemented by plasma screen displays in the modern surgery.

Toys and books in the consulting room help put young patients at their ease, but again they must be safe, clean, and not trip the elderly.

Medical equipment

Accurate scales and height/length measures for babies and older children are vital equipment for all practices, and together with Wright peak flow meters (low reading) and normal range charts should be in every consulting room (Figure 33.1). Paediatric blood

---

ABC of One to Seven, 5th edition. Edited by B. Valman. © 2010 Blackwell Publishing, ISBN: 978-1-4051-8105-1.

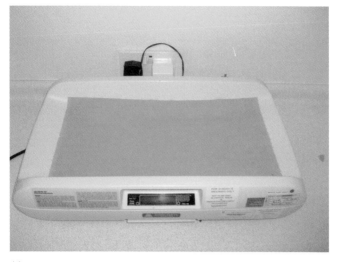

(a)

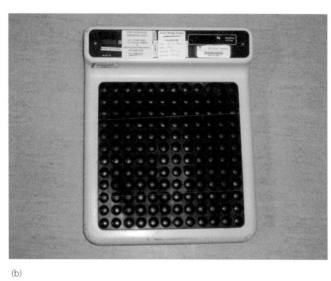

(b)

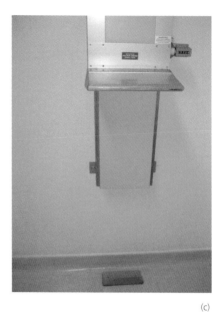

(c)

Figure 33.1 (a) Baby scales. (b) Platform scales. (c) Measuring equipment.

pressure cuffs should be available with the appropriate normal ranges. Demonstration syringe models for parent/teacher training in adrenaline injection are helpful if the practice is competent to train lay personnel.

Child health surveillance equipment should be chosen in conjunction with the local community paediatrician and health visitors to ensure that the professionals using the equipment are trained correctly and measurements are compatible.

The availability of good equipment for minor injuries will prevent children having lengthy unpleasant waits in the local accident and emergency department. Skilled application of tissue glues can often replace the terror and pain of sutures. EMLA cream can reduce the pain of injections.

Home visits and out-of-hours calls

The number of home visits undertaken by GPs halved between 1995 and 2006, and now only 4% of consultations are in the home, mainly for the housebound and very elderly. This means that practices are often dependent on other team members for vital information about family and social circumstances. Even the practice of trying to engage hard-to-reach families through home visiting by midwives and health visitors lacks robust evidence of effectiveness in the UK, although it must be pointed out that such evidence is hard to collect. No longer are GPs obliged to provide 24-hour emergency care for all patients, and accident and emergency departments have been seeing increasing numbers of children with minor illness, who might have been better served by advice from GPs. The range of service providers for out-of-hours care can be confusing for parents, especially those who have recently moved, and it is essential that the practice advertises clearly the process for urgent advice, and organizes fail-safe call diversion. NHS Direct (and NHS 24 in Scotland), cooperatives, commercial deputizing services, walk-in centres, and paediatric assessment units need to network closely with general practices to provide timely shared information about children.

Hospital-at-home services for children are offered in many parts of the country for either acute or continuing care, or both. Close working with general practices is essential for these schemes to work well.

Paediatric emergencies are rare, but it is vitally important that primary care is equipped to deal with them. All practices should have child and infant airways, adrenaline, and dose schedules readily available. GPs should carry with them parenteral penicillin to be given to any child suspected of meningococcal disease before admission to hospital. The system for checking that drugs are in date and replaced must be rigorous, and doctors' bags must be safe from inquisitive children.

The team

The GP is only one member of the PHCT, and Table 33.1 illustrates other team members. Not all these professionals are attached to all practices, and the list is not exclusive, but indicates how children may benefit from the availability of a vast range of skills.

It is essential for the PHCT to meet regularly to exchange information and seek each other's support and advice about the children they are seeing. Best practice consists of semi-formal chaired meetings wherein each case presented for discussion is logged and summarized and action points defined for future reference. Such meetings should aim to break down destructive barriers between different professionals and improve working relationships. It is vital to maintain close trusting relationships with Health Visitors whose work is increasingly based outside the practice.

Table 33.1 Primary health care team members (in addition to general practitioner) and their responsibilities.

Practice nurse	Minor injuries, health education, immunizations
Health visitor	Child health surveillance, immunization, nutritional advice, health education, management of behavioural problems, family nurse partnership projects
Social worker	Advice and support in the management of 'at risk' children, benefits advice, children with special needs, family therapy, and safeguarding against child abuse (including sexual abuse)
Community psychiatric nurse	Emotional disorders and mental illness (liaising with local Child and Adolescent Mental Health Services)
Psychologist	Emotional disorders. Educational problems
Dietitian	Special diets, obesity, food allergy, vegetarian families, diabetic children
Practice manager	Appointments, clinic times, complaints, staff relations
Community nurse	Caring for the seriously ill child at home. Specialist services include Macmillan care

Collaborating around service provision

There is continuing debate around how strong should be the focus on general practice as the central provider of health care for children, and in many parts of the country health visitors are no longer directly attached to practices. Commercially operated polyclinics are strongly resisted by the majority of GPs but there is more productive debate around 'care without walls' collaborations for integrated children's health care.

Children's centres

In most parts of the country there has been little reporting of the impact on primary care for children of this government initiative to build on Sure-start programmes and integrate preschool health, education, and social care provision in children's centres.

In April 2006, statutory Local Safeguarding Children Boards (LSCBs) replaced Area Child Protection Committees (ACPCs) to enhance the safeguarding of children. Most general practice teams have experience of working with designated clinicians and social workers for child protection.

Referrals

Interprofessional and interagency communication is a vital component of effective primary care for children. All communication should include a minimum data set of name, address, telephone number, and date of birth. Table 33.2 is a reminder of other useful information.

Preventive care

Immunization
GPs have to meet immunization targets to receive payments for 'direct enhanced services'. The success of this policy depends not

Table 33.2 Interprofessional communication about a child.

Helpful information for general practice referrals	Helpful information for specialist responses
History of child's complaint	Extra vital information obtained
Relevant family and social history	Diagnosis and treatment plan
Other agencies or professionals	What the family has been told participating in care and their input
Development (if relevant)	Date of planned review (if any)
Present and previously tried medication	If the child has been discharged, the circumstances under which he should be referred again
Allergies and intolerances	
Investigation results	
What the family doctor thinks worries the parents and what is worrying the doctor	

Table 33.3 UK immunization schedule.

Age	Diseases protected against
At birth to babies at high risk	Tuberculosis
At birth to babies born to Hepatitis B positive mothers	Hepatitis B
2 months	Diphtheria, tetanus, pertussis, polio, Hib, pneumococcal infection
3 months	Diphtheria, tetanus, pertussis, polio, Hib, meningitis C
4 months	Diphtheria, tetanus, pertussis, polio, Hib, meningitis C, pneumococcal infection
Around 12 months	Hib, meningitis C
Around 13 months	MMR, pneumococcal infection
3 years and 4 months or soon after (PSB)	Booster diphtheria, tetanus, polio, MMR
10–14 years	BCG (after Heaf test)
15–18 years	Polio, tetanus, diphtheria

Check www.immunisation.nhs.uk/Immunisation_Schedule for updates. BCG, bacille Calmette–Guérin; Hib, *Haemophilus influenzae* type b; MMR, measles, mumps, rubella; PSB, preschool booster.

only on the financial motivation, but also on the defined population of general practices and their unified approach to treatment and prevention.

Each immunization must be performed by a suitably trained member of the team, and records enabling the rapid identification of children with incomplete courses should be kept. Health visitors are ideally trained and situated to optimize vaccine uptake by education and counselling. Table 33.3 shows the schedule, from which it can be seen that the necessary frequent child attendances at the surgery create ideal opportunities for health promotion and surveillance.

Child health surveillance

Practices offering efficient child health surveillance are rewarded under the Quality Outcomes Framework payment scheme, but the payment reflects scant emphasis on this part of GP workload.

The Hall Report in 1989 and subsequent editions of *Health for All Children* resulted in a programme that reduced many specific time-consuming developmental checks and replaced them with a less structured approach that placed greater emphasis on asking parents the correct questions and being more sensitive to parental concern. GPs and health visitors need to have a detailed knowledge of child development. The old rigid system was deemed inappropriate because children do not all develop skills at the same time (Table 33.4). In particular, every opportunity should be taken to advise on accident prevention, behavioural problems, nutrition, and

dental care. A standard form is helpful in collecting data for the child's practice record, parent-held records, and for audit (Box 33.1).

Every Child Matters took record standardization further with proposals for the introduction of a national Common Assessment Framework (CAF) as an important part of a strategy for helping children and young people to achieve the five priority outcomes of:

1 *Being healthy* – enjoying good physical and mental health and living a healthy lifestyle;
2 *Staying safe* – being protected from harm and neglect;
3 *Enjoying and achieving* – getting the most out of life and developing the skills for adulthood;
4 *Making a positive contribution* – being involved with the community and society and not engaging in antisocial or offending behaviour;
5 *Economic well-being* – not being prevented by economic disadvantage from achieving their full potential in life.

There is a long way to go before such a framework is integrated into general practice.

Maintaining evidence-based practice

The 2004 publication of the *National Service Framework for Children, Young People and Maternity Services* has proved fundamental to much of the recent thinking about services for children.

The RCGP Curriculum for Care of Children and Young People highlights key issues for primary care under Standards:

1 Promoting health and well-being;
2 Supporting parenting;
3 Child, young person, and family centred services;
4 Growing up into adulthood; and
5 Safeguarding and promoting the welfare of children and young people.

The pace at which service change is happening and the diversity of primary care practice, as well as the appropriate focus on prioritizing local needs, means that every general practice needs to review and update their services for children on a regular basis. Examples of where recent evidence has changed practice in primary care for children include the following.

- *Screening for postnatal depression* – standardized instruments have some drawbacks connected with parental suspicions and cultural diversity, so that further work is needed to detect and treat this condition which carries serious implications for children.
- *Sudden infant death syndrome* – here current evidence confirms that exposure to smoke, (including sharing a bed with a parent who is a smoker), sharing a bed with a parent who has had alcohol, sleeping prone or with the baby's head covered by bedding are the main avoidable risk factors.
- *Breastfeeding* – there is robust evidence that mothers' choice to breastfeed and successful continuation of feeding can be influenced by interventions in primary care including support groups.

Table 33.4 Ranges of normal developmental abilities. The red line shows the range of ages when normal children start to have that ability. If parents suspect that a child may have delay in an aspect of development, the chart can be used to determine whether all or some abilities fall within the normal range. The child's age is marked at the foot of the chart and by placing a vertical line from that age, the child's abilities can be compared with the normal range.

Developmental check	1 year	18 months	2 years	3 years	4 years	5 years
Physical skills	Walks without help					
	Walks holding furniture	Can kick a ball				
		Walks up steps alone				
	Stands without help	Can throw a ball				
				Can balance on one foot for a second	Can catch a bounced ball	
					Can hop on one leg	
Manual dexterity	Can pick up a small object		Can draw straight lines			
		Can build a tower of 4 bricks				
	likes to scribble			Can copy a circle	Can copy a square	
					Can draw a rudimentary person	
Vision, hearing, and speech		Can point to parts of the body		Can talk in full sentences		
		Can put two words together		Knows first and second names		
		Starts to learn single words		Can name a colour	Can define seven words	
Social behaviour and play		Can eat with a spoon and fork			Can eat with a knife and fork	
	Copies housework	Can undress without help		Can dress without help		
	Can drink from a cup	Stays dry in day		Stays dry at night		
Age (months)	12 13 14 15 16 17 18 19 20 21 22 23 24			36	48	60
Age (years)	1		2	3	4	5

Box 33.1 **Standard form for collecting data at 4.0–4.5 years.**

Review at 4 – 4½ years
For parent to complete

Health Topics for discussion: Tick ☑	Accident prevention ▪ Developmental needs in school ▪ Prevention of head lice, threadworms, etc. ▪

Does your child have any problems which may affect schooling?   Yes / no / not sure
If 'Yes' or 'not sure' please say what the problem is _____

Does your child have any problems with movement and / or coordination?   Yes / no / not sure
If 'Yes' or 'not sure' please say what the problem is _____

Is your child clean and dry during the day and night?   Yes / no / not sure
If 'Yes' or 'not sure' please say what the problem is _____

Does your child wheeze or have a night cough?   Yes / no / not sure
Do you have any worries about your child's health?   Yes / no / not sure
If 'Yes' or 'not sure' please say what the problem is _____

Do you have any worries about your child's behaviour?   Yes / no / not sure
If 'Yes' or 'not sure' please say what the problem is _____

Comments _____

Which school is your child likely to attend? _____
Are your child's immunisations up to date including the preschool booster? Yes / no
Top Copy: Stay in Record Pink Copy: to School Nurse

Review at 4 – 4½ years
¥ Please place a sticker (if available) otherwise write in space

Surname
First names
NHS number   Local no
Address _____
Postcode _____   Sex   M/F
   D.O.B. __/__/__
G.P.   Code
H.V.   Code

Further comments on consultation sheet: YES/NO
Date of Examination ___/___/___
Age in years _____
Name of Examiner
Examinar Code Number   Examination centre
HEIGHT   cms   centile
WEIGHT   kg   centile

Any previous ongoing medical problems? No ☐   Yes ☐
If 'yes' please specify   (1) _____ (2) _____ (3) _____
ICD Code

ITEM	GUIDE TO CONTENT	CODE (Ring one)*	COMMENT
Physical	Not examined routinely.	S P O T R N	
Vision	Not examined routinely.	S P O T R N	
Hearing	Not examined routinely.	S P O T R N	
Locomotion	Not examined routinely.	S P O T R N	
Manipulation	Not examined routinely.	S P O T R N	
Speech Lang.	Not examined routinely.	S P O T R N	
Behaviour	Not examined routinely.	S P O T R N	
Testes	ring 'N' for girl	S P O T R N	
Heart		S P O T R N	

* (If one or more codes seem to apply select the last one e.g. R takes priority over T, T over O etc.)
S = Satisfactory (normal result)
P = Problem (signficant condition record)
O = Observation (special recall arranged)
T = Treatment or investigation underway
R = Referred to any community or hospital service
N = Not examined for this item
Copy: Stay in Record

Referred to (1) _____ (2) _____
(3) _____
Special recall in _____ wks/mths
Signature

Further reading

Hall D. Elliman D. *Health for All Children*, 4th edn. Oxford University Press, Oxford, 2006.

Guidelines to access in mid-consultation

The most helpful collection is that of the Royal College of Paediatrics and Child Health. http://www.rcpch.ac.uk/Research/CE/Guidelines/national-guidelines

Web references

Children's centres: http://www.standards.dfes.gov.uk/primary/faqs/foundation_stage/1162267/

Safeguarding: http://www.everychildmatters.gov.uk/socialcare/safeguarding/lscb/

National Framework: http://www.dh.gov.uk/PolicyAndGuidance/HealthAndSocialCareTopics/ChildrenServices/ChildrenServicesInformation/ChildrenServicesInformationArticle/fs/en?CONTENT_ID=4089111&chk=U8Ecln

Every Child Matters: www.everychildmatters.gov.uk

Children Act 2004: http://www.opsi.gov.uk/acts/acts2004/20040031.htm

National Screening Committee Children's sub-group: http://www.nsc.nhs.uk/ch_screen/child_ind.htm

RCGP Curriculum: http://www.rcgp-curriculum.org.uk/PDF/curr_8_Care_of_Children_and_Young_People.pdf

CHAPTER 34

Services for Children: The Community

Arlene Boroda

North West London NHS Trust, London, UK

OVERVIEW

- Most health care for children is delivered outside the hospital.
- The child's needs should determine where the health service is delivered.
- Effective services require the close liaison of all agencies including health, social care, and education supporting and enabling parents.
- Child health is targeted at vulnerable groups such as the homeless, asylum seekers, new arrivals to an area, and continued health promotion and advice.
- Statutory work includes immunizations, child protection, and educational paediatrics.

Primary and secondary care services

Services are provided by:
- The primary care service and is universal; and
- The child health service, which is a secondary care service and provides specialist care for children with problems.

Primary health care

The round the clock health care to ill children at home and within the community is largely provided by general practitioners (GPs) and the primary health care team. Appropriately trained primary health care practitioners provide child health surveillance, child health promotion, and accident prevention. This service may be provided within the GP practices, within clinics, and increasingly within child centres and polyclinics. The supervising clinician may be a child health consultant paediatrician or a GP with a special interest in paediatrics. The clinics are well placed to meet the health needs of vulnerable children including the following:
- Families not registered with a GP;
- Mobile families;
- Immigrant families, homeless, or refugees; and
- Families whose GPs do not carry out surveillance.

Computers in child health

Provider units have a child health computer system. The computer modules include: a child register with neonatal data, immunizations, preschool and school health modules, special needs register, and child protection data. The systems can store basic child health data, allocate health visitors, generate appointments for immunizations, and child health surveillance (Table 34.1). Schedules of children due for screening may be produced. Data may be used for public health analysis and audit.

Personal child health record

The personal child health record is a manual record held by the parents. This is intended to be a complete record of the child's health. If completed by all health professionals at all contacts it may become a record of child health data, immunizations, child health surveillance, and GP and health visitor visits. It has advice on child growth and development and growth charts.

Child health service

This service includes:
- Surveillance of growth, health, and development;
- Enabling and parent support;
- Prevention of illness, poor health, and accidents by health promotion and immunization;
- Advice to parents and carers about common children's health issues;
- Medical assessment of children thought to have been abused or neglected;
- Identification of 'children in need' of services and children who have been abused – Children Act 1989; and
- Identification and assessment of children with special educational needs – Education Act 1996.

The child health programme is shown in Table 34.1.

Doctors and nurses in community child health

The medical team is usually led by a consultant paediatrician, either based in a hospital or a community setting. Increasingly, the consultants are contracted to work in both the acute services as well as the community services, providing an integrated model of care

ABC of One to Seven, 5th edition. Edited by B. Valman. © 2010 Blackwell Publishing, ISBN: 978-1-4051-8105-1.

Table 34.1 The child health programme.

Age	Examiner	Procedure	Health promotion
Neonatal	GP or hospital doctor	Physical examination (including height, weight, skull circumference, heart, hips, eyes for red reflex, genitalia)	Feeding and nutrition Baby care – sleeping position Sibling management Transport in a car Effects of smoking
	Midwife	Screening for phenylketonuria, cystic fibrosis, hypothyroidism, haemoglobinopathy, MCADD	
	Audiologist	Hearing test	
Within 14 days	Health visitor	General health check of newborn Screen for jaundice	Feeding advice Baby care advice
6–8 weeks	Doctor	Physical examination: height, weight, skull circumference Heart, eyes, genitalia	Immunization Recognition of illness Nutrition – promotion of breastfeeding Activities to aid development Dangers: fire, scalds, falls, overheating
7–9 months	Health visitor	Targeted hearing tests – distraction test Assess for squint Assess for growth and development	Accident prevention; choking, scalds, safety in cars and house, sunburn Dental prophylaxis Developmental needs Nutrition
2-year contact	Health visitor	Assessment of health and development by history and observation Consider if child has SEN and notify LEA Complete CAF – assess child's needs	Accident prevention: falls from heights, road safety, and ingestion of poisons Developmental needs Mixing with children – mother and baby groups Management of behaviour
Vulnerable children (asylum seekers), new arrivals in borough	Health visitor/school nurse	Assess development by history and observation Check height, weight, skull circumference Check vision Complete CAF	Immunization Accident prevention Nutrition Advice on local services
5+	School nurse	Information received from health visitor and preschool records Tests vision Checks weight and height Meets parents Checks immunization status Requires parental consent to see child Consider if child has SEN and notify LEA Complete CAF	Refers to GP for missed immunizations
	School nurse/audiologist	Tests hearing – sweep pure tone	
Any age	School nurse/paediatrician	Assess children at request of parents, school, school nurse and a health professional Refer to therapists and specialist services Requires parental consent to see child	Health advice Advice on local services
13+	School nurse	Drop-in sessions for young people Immunizations – new vaccines	Health promotion and advice National programs
15+	School nurse	Immunizations	

CAF, common assessment framework; LEA, local education authority; MCADD, medium chain acyl CoA dehydrogenase deficiency; SEN, special educational needs.

and training for junior staff, putting the child's needs as the centre of where the service is best delivered. The training of specialists may produce a specialist in community paediatrics, neurodisability, audiological medicine, public health, and emotional and behavioural problems. Service delivery may be managed according to geographical area or by conditions.

Health visitors

Health visitors are specialist nurses with obstetric and paediatric training in children from birth to school entry. They provide advice and support to pregnant mothers and then continue this education and practical hands on monitoring of the children until they hand over the case to the child's school nurse. Increasingly, their work is with targeted families such as child protection, premature babies, low birth weight babies, and vulnerable families such as mothers with mental health problems or those who are teenage parents.

Health visitors see all children who transfer into their area and send a copy of their assessment to the local child health computer system. They also pick up cases that have missed their newborn screening programs and arrange for these tests to be performed.

Specialist nurse teams

Specialist nurses lead teams in the following disciplines:
- Domestic violence;
- Breastfeeding;
- Homeless families and refugees;
- Teenage pregnancy;
- Counselling for haemoglobinopathies;
- Attention deficit hyperactivity disorder (ADHD);
- Incontinence services;
- Child protection and safeguarding children;
- Epilepsy and disability;
- Looked after children – children in the care of the local authority: Children Act 1989 S20 or S31; and
- Care of the vulnerable newborn infant at home.

School health service

Educational medicine is the study and practice of child health and paediatrics in relation to the process of learning. It includes child development, the educational setting, the child's responses to school, the disorders that interfere with a child's capacity to learn, and needs of disabled children (Figure 34.1). The team work closely with teachers, psychologists, and others working with the child, understanding the influences of the family and the social environment. Each service provider has a named doctor for education, who links with the therapist and the lead for education.

Routine health assessments have been discontinued. The school health program offers selective paediatric assessments for children with school-based problems and other special health needs. The school nurse provides the link between the education services and specialist paediatric assessments.

School nurse

School nurses are involved in health promotion for children, parents, and education staff. All children entering school will be overseen by a school nurse, who has taken over the child's care from the health visitor.

School nurses provide the link between teachers and specialist health services as they are in the schools and meet with school staff, talk to the parents, and have seen the child on school entry. They identify problems such as general health issues, development, behaviour, and social concerns.

Children within the child protection system are monitored by the school health team who have a case load. School nurses have specialist training in this area. Nursing assistants perform the weight and height checks.

Children with special needs

Special needs include speech, language and communication, behaviour, learning, mobility, sensory, and emotional difficulties (see Chapter 29). Behavioural problems, social deprivation, homelessness, and substance misuse emphasize the close working with social care and child psychiatry.

Education Act 1996

If a child's needs cannot be met by the resources and facilities of a school, then a statutory assessment by the agencies supporting the child is carried out to formulate a Statement of Special Educational Needs. The views of educational professionals, health team, and parents are sought. The medical advice involves an assessment by a paediatrician who will refer to the reports carried out by the therapists, the parents, and the psychologists. The parents and the local education authority advise on a school placement. Increasingly, children with special needs are placed in mainstream schools. However, specialist schools are available for physically disabled children, those with severe learning disabilities, and children with emotional and behavioural problems.

Further reading

Hall D, Elliman D. *Health for All Children*, 4th edn. Oxford University Press, Oxford, 2002.
Polnoy L. *Community Paediatrics*, 3rd edn. Churchill Livingstone, 2002.

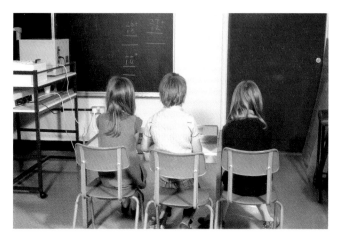

Figure 34.1 School health service.

CHAPTER 35

Services for Children: Outpatient Clinics and Day-Care

Bernard Valman

Northwick Park Hospital and Imperial College London, UK

OVERVIEW

- If children are to receive appropriate health care they need a range of connected services: primary care from general practice and secondary care through the community child heath service and the hospital.
- The hospital provides outpatient, day, emergency, ambulatory, and inpatient services.
- Services in the outpatient clinics and day-care unit are described in this chapter and emergency, ambulatory, and inpatient services are discussed in Chapter 36.

Outpatient consultation

An efficient receptionist is the pivot of the clinic. She should like children and have sympathy with their mothers. She will be the first person to meet the family on arrival and her kindness will affect their feelings about the unit (Figure 35.1). A paediatric nurse measures and weighs the children and collects urine specimens if there is a specific indication. In most cases the doctor can examine the child with only the mother present.

An average-sized unit cannot manage more than about 2000 new outpatients and 8000 return visits a year. Ideally, all children should be seen within a week of referral, but reasonable targets are that urgent cases are seen within a week, 'soon' cases within 4 weeks, and routine cases within 6 weeks. The referral letter should describe the parents' and doctor's worries, current medication, investigations performed, and the family or social background. Referral letters are read by the consultant, who determines the date of the appointment according to the probable diagnosis. If the letter is illegible or vital information is missing a dangerous delay may occur before the child is seen. Packing the clinic with spuriously urgent cases may prevent any child from having an adequate consultation. Some patients book the appointment time online with the 'choose and book' procedure, but a referral letter from the family doctor is still needed.

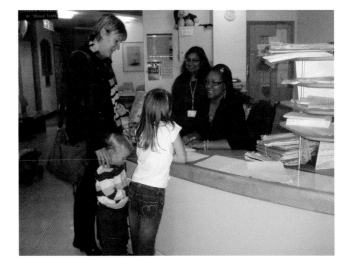

Figure 35.1 Reception.

New patients are usually seen by a consultant or by a specialist registrar who discusses the child with the consultant. Parents need to know that not every child can see the consultant, or fewer patients would be seen. Most parents prefer to see the same doctor each time. Considerable paediatric experience is needed before outpatient care can be provided competently and junior staff should be supervised by a consultant.

Indications for referral

Families may pressurize a general practitioner (GP) to seek a second opinion even though he does not consider it necessary. Most GPs will anticipate the parents' feelings and arrange a consultation at a suitable stage. There is usually no hesitation in referring children when the diagnosis is obscure, a particular consultant has special expertise in that problem, the disease is likely to cause long-term disability, special investigations are necessary, or the advice of a large team is appropriate. The decision is harder when the consultant is unlikely to be able to provide additional treatment, but the parents may be helped to accept their doctor's explanation and management after being seen in hospital. For example, the parents of a child with recurrent upper respiratory infections may imagine that he has a serious disease and be reassured by an independent opinion.

ABC of One to Seven, 5th edition. Edited by B. Valman. © 2010 Blackwell Publishing, ISBN: 978-1-4051-8105-1.

Type of problem seen

The most common problems in new patients include recurrent respiratory tract infections, bronchial asthma, behavioural problems, enuresis, failure to thrive and growth problems, recurrent abdominal pain, and convulsions. Children with systolic murmurs are referred directly to a paediatric cardiologist after the murmur has been detected at routine examinations, and children with recurrent urinary tract infections are often sent for further investigations.

Some chronic conditions are followed up in hospital clinics because their management demands special skill. Joint clinics may be held with specialists in diabetes, haematology, orthopaedics, or plastic surgery, and there may be special clinics for cystic fibrosis, gastroenterology, fits, or chronic handicaps. Children with severe asthma tend to be seen in general paediatric clinics or an asthma clinic as they form the largest single group of children with a recurring or persisting disability. Community child health services provide clinics in neurodevelopmental disability, behavioural problems, hearing impairment, enuresis, and attention deficit hyperactivity disorder.

Appropriate referrals

Children with suspected diabetes mellitus or with features suggesting non-accidental injury should be discussed with the admitting registrar immediately; in these circumstances an outpatient referral is dangerous. Similarly, children with an acute illness of unknown cause may well have recovered by the time of the appointment.

Neonatal follow-up clinics

Most special care baby units arrange to follow up-selected patients until they are 18 months or 2 years old. Most were born weighing under 1500 g and some had birth asphyxia or less common problems such as neonatal convulsions. These infants are usually seen at a separate clinic, where enough time is available for developmental assessment.

Appointment systems and accommodation

There are several problems with appointment systems; ensuring that new patients are given enough time for their consultation and that there is an allowance for patients who arrive late or default or for those with complex problems that take a long time to deal with. Children become irritable and hungry if they have to wait too long and their mothers may forget their main problems when they finally enter the consulting room.

The outpatient department for children should be designed especially for them (Figure 35.2). There should be a separate waiting area with furniture of the appropriate size and no stairs, lifts, or heavy doors, which could cause accidents. Rooms are needed for measuring, changing, breastfeeding, and urine collection, and the consulting room needs toys and books, pictures on the walls and ceiling, and a small table and chair for toddlers.

Communication

A letter sent promptly to the GP should contain the probable diagnosis, management, and prognosis. The history and physical findings should be noted briefly. The results of investigations can be included in a second letter to the GP with a copy to the parents.

Indications for day-care

Day-care is the best method of providing certain services, and although the cost needs to be considered it should not be the main reason for advocating day-care. Day patients are those who attend for observation, investigation, surgery, or other treatment and who need some form of supervision or period of recovery (Box 35.1). The children are not separated from their parents, they sleep at

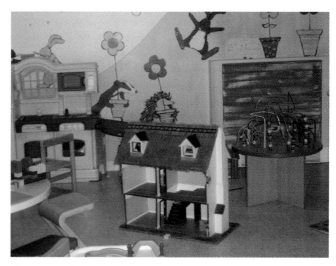

Figure 35.2 Play area.

Box 35.1 **Day care procedures**

Investigations
- Urine collection:
  - clean catch
  - suprapubic puncture
  - catheter
- Blood test
- Sweat test
- Food tolerance test
- Isotope renal scan
- Micturating cystourethrogram
- Endoscopy

Treatment
- Surgical
  - grommets
  - hernia
  - circumcision
  - dental
- Chemotherapy
- Blood transfusion

home at night, and the life of the family is less disrupted than if they were admitted. Parents usually prefer to bring their children to a day centre, if necessary more than once, than have them admitted. In some busy departments day-care may be the only way of ensuring that there are enough beds and nurses for all the children who need admission.

About one-third of all elective general surgery in children can be carried out in a day unit. Suitable surgical problems include aspiration of the middle ear and grommet insertion, hernia operations, circumcision, and endoscopy. There is also a place for preventive and restorative dental care, particularly in disabled children. If the mother has satisfactory postoperative analgesics to give her child at home, these procedures are as safe in a day unit as in an inpatient ward. Postoperative visits or phone calls to the home by doctors or nurses are rarely necessary. The anaesthetic given must be suitable for day-care, and the surgery should not be delegated to a junior doctor.

Indications for medical day-care are less well defined, and the patients being seen need to be reviewed regularly to avoid overwhelming the service. The main indications are investigations, or repeated chemotherapy for leukaemia or other malignancies. Children with failure to thrive or developmental delay, who were previously admitted for long periods, can be investigated completely in a day-care unit.

Day-care can complement an outpatient visit, especially with necessary but difficult investigations. Taking blood from a kicking, fat toddler can be an ordeal for everyone in a hectic outpatient clinic; in the day-care unit it may be much easier especially if there is time for an anaesthetic cream to become effective. Some tests, such as sweat tests or food tolerance tests, take a long time but the day-care unit's playroom reduces the ordeal. Toddlers are often distressed by a renal scan and even more by a micturating cystogram, but preliminary sedation in the day-care unit and a bed to sleep in afterwards may reduce the anxiety and discomfort.

CHAPTER 36

Services for Children: Emergency, Ambulatory, and Inpatients

Bernard Valman

Northwick Park Hospital and Imperial College London, UK

OVERVIEW

- Parents of an ill child may find it difficult to determine whether they should call an ambulance, take their child to the nearest emergency department of a hospital, phone their general practitioner (GP), or manage the child at home without medical advice (Figure 36.1).

- Parents will be helped to make this decision by books written for this purpose or by contacting NHS Direct by phone or online (see Further reading at the end of this chapter).

- Ideally, there should be a separate paediatric emergency department. If it is sited next to the adult unit some resources can be shared.

- Ambulatory care and acute assessment units reduce the need for admission.

- Inpatient units need child-centred buildings with facilities for mothers to stay next to their children.

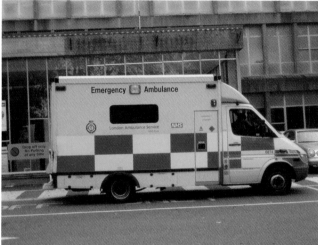

Figure 36.1 Parents may have difficulty in determining whether urgent attention is needed.

Emergency department

Until recently this was called the accident and emergency department. Ideally, there should be a separate paediatric emergency department with a separate waiting room, consulting rooms, and drug cupboard. Equipment of appropriate size for varying ages can only be available easily if a resuscitation room is equipped specifically for children. If there is no specific paediatric emergency department, a section of the main department can be designated for children. Where emergencies in children are usually managed in the main department, there is the disadvantage that about three-quarters of the patients are adults and few of the nursing and medical staff has any postgraduate paediatric training.

A triage nurse sees the child shortly after arrival to ensure that severely ill children are seen by a doctor immediately. In most hospitals a member of the paediatric team is on call to give a second opinion to the emergency staff.

In many inner city areas the emergency department provides a great deal of primary care, particularly in the evenings and at weekends. If the paediatric junior staff on call spend most of their time giving primary care they may find it difficult to fulfil their other commitments, which may include the care of severely ill children.

Ambulatory paediatrics

Ambulatory paediatrics describes a philosophy lying behind the provision of care and does not form a specialty of paediatrics. In many countries the term is used to describe the full range of care not involving inpatient practice, and frequently includes primary care. In the UK, ambulatory paediatrics includes the assessment and treatment of acutely ill children attending hospital. Some of these children may be observed for short periods, often only for a few hours. Some hospitals have specific units for ambulatory care while others have combined the service with the paediatric emergency department.

The paediatric and child health services aim to provide care without hospital admission whenever possible, and when admission is essential aim to reduce the duration to a minimum. To provide this service considerable flexibility is needed to meet the needs of parents and children and the geographical characteristics of the population. Acute assessment services form part of the integrated child health service. Home care, community children's nursing, and

---

ABC of One to Seven, 5th edition. Edited by B. Valman. © 2010 Blackwell Publishing, ISBN: 978-1-4051-8105-1.

arrangements for review by paediatricians are essential components of the service.

Acute assessment unit

The aim of the unit is to provide a rapid specialist consultation for acutely ill children in support of primary care services. In some hospitals it is called the paediatric emergency department and in others the paediatric ambulatory care unit. The assessment of an acute illness in a child frequently requires a period of observation, with access to investigations such as pathology and imaging, suitable monitoring equipment, and specialist nurses. Facilities should be adequate for resuscitation and stabilization of critically ill children needing airway support, ventilation, and intravenous fluids. These are the equivalent of care provided in inpatient facilities. The distinction of this group of children from those who would be classified as inpatient admissions is not well defined, other than by duration of stay. Such units aim to prevent admission where possible and when it proves necessary, to shorten the stay to the minimum required for safe management of the illness. The decision to discharge a child should be taken by a senior experienced paediatrician. Some children assessed in the unit will need transfer to inpatient beds.

In acute paediatric practice a home care nursing team is likely to reduce length of stay and for a minority of patients may prevent admission. It may also prevent the admission of children with chronic illness and disability. It is essential that the unit should be supported by a paediatric home care nursing team.

The costs of care in this type of unit are equivalent to those of inpatient episodes. The development of these units is primarily for quality purposes and to manage the child for as short a period as possible within the hospital and to promote early discharge for care at home by parents, rather than for reducing cost. Although there may be a reduction in numbers of inpatient bed days, an increased number of paediatric acute episodes are likely to occur.

Admission to hospital

Children need nurses and ancillary staff attuned to their needs to prevent unnecessary distress. Although the admission of a mother with the child may reduce this trauma, in some units mothers are daunted by the unwelcoming attitudes of staff and by primitive accommodation.

Teenagers need staff and facilities that are different to those for younger children and adults. Their problems range from motorcycle accidents in boys, gynaecological problems in girls, and drug-related problems in both sexes. A separate annexe to the children's ward could provide this service, but it is difficult to attract staff with the appropriate skills. Teenagers over the age of 15 years are usually admitted to adult wards.

Indications for admission

The severely ill child clearly needs to be admitted. Children with problems needing admission include those with fractures requiring operation or traction and those with suspected acute appendicitis.

Some children need urgent medical investigations and nursing observation and others have urgent social and medical reasons such as non-accidental injuries. Some medical patients need nursing and treatment that cannot be provided at home, such as intravenous fluids for gastroenteritis and tube feeding for bronchiolitis. Complex problems may need the opinions of several specialists, who may be better coordinated by a short admission, although most investigations can now be performed in a day-care unit. Severely ill children needing intensive monitoring or ventilation are usually nursed in the intensive care unit, managed jointly by the paediatrician and anaesthetist in charge of the unit, or may need to be transferred to a paediatric intensive care unit if facilities are not available on site.

Admission procedure

When direct admission is sought the GP usually discusses the problem with the paediatric specialist registrar. This telephone conversation helps to clarify the problem and decide whether there are any special social reasons contributing to the admission. Arrangements can also be discussed for a possible early discharge or ways of avoiding admission. The average length of stay for paediatric inpatients is about 2 days, but if beds are to be available for every admission requested the average occupancy cannot exceed 70%. This means that during epidemics patients may have to be discharged sooner than usual and followed up in the ambulatory care unit or outpatient clinic.

Common reasons for admission

The sudden deterioration that may occur in infants with bronchiolitis or severe asthma has encouraged GPs to send these patients to hospital (Box 36.1). Some of these children could be nursed at home if the GP or community paediatric nursing staff visited them often enough to admit them if they deteriorated. However, GPs are under pressure from parents to admit children to hospital. Such expectations are hard to resist and children may be admitted to an assessment bed in the ambulatory care unit and transferred to the inpatient ward for a short period during the acute phase of the illness. Children with a first febrile convulsion may be admitted to exclude meningitis and to allay the parents' fears.

The introduction of effective drugs has persuaded parents that they do not have to wait a week for the natural history of an asthmatic attack to take place. Many units now have an open house system so that a child with a severe attack can be seen in the ambulatory care unit and be admitted if the attack is not quickly relieved. This early treatment may result in more children being seen in the ambulatory care unit; they have symptoms for a shorter period and miss less school. Repeated admissions also indicate

---

Box 36.1 **Admission**

- Surgery
- Urgent investigations
- Nursing
- Complex problems

that the management is ineffective and needs to be changed. Most medical investigations and about one-third of paediatric surgery can now be carried out in a day-care unit.

Nurses in paediatric wards

The shift system results in each child being nursed by six to eight different nurses each week, despite the fact that each nurse may look after the same group of children each time she is on duty. The mother is therefore the only person who can provide continuity of care for a child, and the admission of the child without the mother is likely to aggravate any feeding or behavioural problems.

Mothers

The attitudes of staff towards mothers determine whether mothers want to stay. The ward sister will set an example and show that they are complementary to the nurses and not usurping the nurses' role. The resident mother needs basic comforts including a folding bed, a cupboard for her clothes, a bathroom, and a room where she can chat to other mothers. She needs to know where to find linen, make tea, and obtain a meal. A list of guidelines will give her more confidence. Some prefer to go home for short periods, especially in the evenings, and they should be encouraged to do so. If a mother does not want to stay in the unit she should not be pressed. Healthy siblings can stay with the patient and mother. More than half of mothers will stay with their children if they are given the opportunity, and this should not be related to the child's age. Most anaesthetists allow the mother to go with the child to the anaesthetic room.

In the ward the mother can carry out the usual care, including feeding, changing, and bathing. She can also take the child for investigations and can keep fluid charts, collect urine, and in some cases observe the flow of intravenous fluids. Selected mothers can be taught simple nursing procedures such as temperature recording and tube feeding. During admission the mother learns more about nursing a sick child and gains confidence (Figure 36.2). The nurses can assess the mother's competence in managing and attitude towards the child and find it easier to assess the appropriate time for discharge. Student nurses may learn a great deal from an experienced mother about the skilled and sensitive care of a young child.

Play is a child's work, not simply amusement. A skilled play leader can help the children to play out the events of the admission, by allowing them to handle syringes and other equipment, and can discover with the mother how the child feels. A child can be introduced to the prospect of surgery by appropriate play. Most wards have a part-time or full-time schoolteacher.

Staff strain

If the admissions policy is working well most of the children on the ward are acutely ill. Many are discharged shortly after they begin to improve so the wards no longer have convalescent patients. The short period of admission and the high discharge rate for each bed produce continuous emotional strains on nursing, junior medical, and secretarial staff. The high rate of admissions is similar to that in an intensive care unit, but the allocation of nurses does not usually take this into account. Staff morale and quality of care can easily fall when nursing and medical staff are working continuously under high pressure. Many units do not have the funds to bring the nursing establishment up to an adequate level and others would find it difficult to recruit enough nurses even if funds were available. Providing more day and community care is often the only solution compatible with providing a continuous service to the child community.

Infectious diseases

The most common infectious disease requiring admission is acute gastroenteritis. Most children with acute gastroenteritis can be managed at home, but those requiring intravenous fluids or those with poor social conditions may need admission. Ideally, these children should be nursed in an annexe to the children's wards. Properly designed cubicles with double doors allow barrier nursing and help to prevent cross-infection (Figure 36.3). Unless the

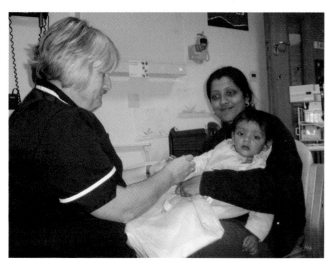

Figure 36.2 The presence of the mother reassures the child.

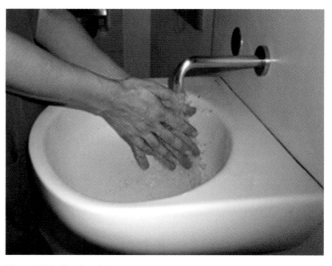

Figure 36.3 Handwashing.

mother is admitted with the child, emotional and social isolation is an inevitable consequence of the physical isolation. Children with measles, chickenpox, mumps, or scarlet fever rarely need to be admitted, although they may be severely ill for a short part of the disease. Children with heavily infected eczema and those with leukaemia who have developed chickenpox are best managed in a barrier-nursed cubicle on a children's ward.

Preparation for admission to the paediatric unit

An admission booklet prepares the mother and child for what they can expect in the ward. Several of these booklets are specially prepared with children in mind and include pictures which they can colour in before arrival. For planned admissions the child can be shown round the ward after finishing the outpatient consultation. As a large proportion of the child population will be admitted or seen at hospital at some stage, a few schools arrange trips to the local hospital. There are now several excellent books written for children about hospital, and the mother can inform herself about ward life as she reads about it to the child.

The newborn

The largest number of infants in hospital are newborn infants, who may account for 5000 admissions a year, compared with 2000 in the paediatric wards. Most of these babies are completely well and in many units they stay next to their mothers throughout the 24 hours. The length of stay depends on the policy of the unit, but most babies are discharged between 6 and 24 hours after birth. During their stay infants should be examined at least once by a member of the paediatric staff and in some units will also be examined by the obstetric junior staff. The mother is taught to care for her infant mainly by the midwife in the antenatal and neonatal period.

About 15% of newborn infants need special nursing care. Most of these infants weigh less than 2000 g at birth, are preterm, have had perinatal asphyxia, or have respiratory problems. Some have feeding difficulties or need phototherapy. To avoid separating all these infants from their mothers some units have provided an 'intermediate' ward, which is a postnatal ward with nurses who can provide simple forms of neonatal special care. This can reduce the number of infants going to the intensive neonatal care unit from 15% to 7%.

A new mother may be frightened and bewildered by the complicated equipment and the appearance of the baby; she may be

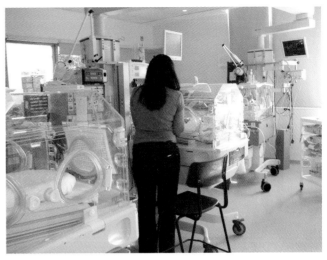

Figure 36.4 Visiting the newborn in the neonatal intensive care unit may be daunting to a parent.

helped by a preliminary explanation from a member of the medical or nursing staff before she enters the unit (Figure 36.4). This explanation can be amplified by a pamphlet. If nursing staff welcome the mother she will not be afraid to visit the unit frequently to touch, change, feed, and later breastfeed her infant. Brothers and sisters should visit the baby from shortly after birth, and a suitable play area with toys will be needed. The social worker to the unit will offer to see the parents individually or in a group to try to reduce stress.

Some units (regional intensive care units) receive babies of extremely low birth weight and those needing artificial ventilation. An increasing number of mothers are transferred to these units before delivery to avoid transporting a sick infant. Separation of a mother from her family may be unavoidable and visiting difficult because of the distance and cost.

Nurses may find it stressful to work in such a unit, especially at night, when staff shortages are common. The design of units with large windows so that the staff can see the sunrise, trees, and birds may reduce this feeling of isolation. The neonatal unit often has a separate establishment of nurses who do not work in any other part of the hospital.

Further reading

Valman B. *When Your Child is Ill: A Home Guide for Parents*, 3rd edn. Dorling Kindersley, London, 2008.
NHS Direct: Tel: 0845 4647. www.nhsdirect.nhs.uk

CHAPTER 37

Audit in Primary Care Paediatrics

Ed Peile

University of Warwick, Coventry, UK

OVERVIEW

- Audit is an important skill for all general practitioners (GPs) involved in the care of children and young people.

- The objective for audit is quality improvement – intelligently auditing and reauditing the services for children will contribute to improved care.

- The process of audit is well defined and easy to follow.

The Royal College of General Practitioners Curriculum for Care of Children and Young People defines as a learning outcome that practitioners should be able to:

- Describe the principles of clinical governance.

- Clinical governance systems do not always recognize children and young people as a separate and vulnerable client group. It is essential that the care of children and young people is given a specific focus within the clinical governance of primary care.

- The components of clinical governance strategies in primary care will include: the safety of treatment and care; safeguarding; the use of evidence-based practice; clinical audit; effective prescribing and referrals; and continuing professional development.

Audit is the name given to the process of assuring the quality of the care that we deliver as health professionals. When we audit any aspect of our care we go through a series of steps, as follows:

1 *What are we doing?* Here we measure our actual performance. For example, what percentage of our asthmatic children have had a peak flow recorded in the past 6 months (Figure 37.1)?

2 *What should we be doing?* Here we decide what standard of care we should be aiming at. This step usually involves consensus among colleagues and reading recent publications.

3 *Comparing points 1 and 2.* Here we face up to how far short of our own standards we actually fall. Sometimes we are pleasantly surprised to find that we have reached them.

4 *Negotiating change.* At this stage we examine, with other relevant health professionals, the facets of our practice that need to be changed to allow us to get nearer to the standard that we have set.

ABC of One to Seven, 5th edition. Edited by B. Valman. © 2010 Blackwell Publishing, ISBN: 978-1-4051-8105-1.

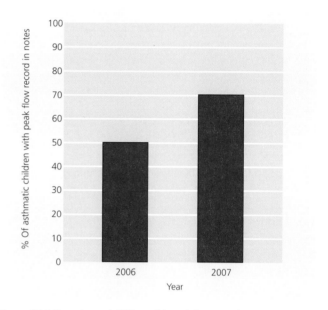

Figure 37.1 Percentage of children with peak flow record in notes.

5 *Closing the loop.* This is a vital step. It entails reauditing the results to see whether our changes have been instituted and whether they are working (Box 37.1). This has to be done over again until the team is satisfied that points 1 and 2 are as close as possible.

Why audit

It is one thing to know what to do, but another to be sure that we are doing it. Audit allows us to see how near we get to our standards. Even better, it shows us how our systems and everyday practice let us down and gives us the opportunity to change them to allow our efforts to be optimized. Audit puts the control of the quality of our work into our own hands.

What to audit?

Medical care should be acceptable, accessible, effective, equitable, and efficient. If we wish to ensure quality then, with this in mind, we should look at what we are doing. This especially applies to the way we manage the common chronic illnesses. When we start to

Box 37.1 **Data collection sheet**

```
                ASTHMA AUDIT PROTOCOL
                 DATA COLLECTION SHEET
     (Please tick when present in notes)

                Emergency   Prescribed  Peak expiratory  Diagnosis
                admissions  broncho-    flow readings    of asthma
 No Patient name in past year dilators  in past year     in notes
  1
  2
  3
  4
  5
  6
  7
  8
  9
 10
 11
 12
 13
 14

 28
 29
 30
 Total:
```

Box 37.2 **Essential equipment**

- Notes (in order)
- Age/sex register (manual or computerized)
- Disease register (manual or computerized)
- Time (staff or your own)
- Sample size graph (Fig. 37.2)

- *Standards and criteria.* These should be explicitly set out and explained and justified.
- *Method.* The actual nuts and bolts of how the audit is going to be performed should be written here. Doing this will clarify the roles of different members of the team doing the audit.
- *Data collection sheet.* A data collection sheet should be designed. This will make it easy for the data to be collected accurately and comprehensively. It will also make totting up results easier.
- *Summary sheet.* This is simply to record the total results.
- *Action and review.* This section needs to be completed at the end of the study. It documents what action is to be taken as a result of the audit and when the audit cycle is to be rerun to gauge the effectiveness of any changes.

look at what we are doing in this way it soon becomes apparent that we could look at the quality of our equipment and buildings (structure), the quality of our treatments and diagnoses and doctor–patient communication, our team working (process), or the quality of our success in preventing the suffering of illness (outcome).

Definitions

Two other terms are crucial to understanding audit:
- *Standard* – This refers to the level of care that we have decided is desirable to achieve. For example, in the care of asthmatic children we may think that we would be satisfied if no more than 3 days of school a year were missed because of asthma. This is our standard.
- *Criterion* – This refers to the element of care to which we are applying our standard. In the above example 'days off school' is a criterion that we are using to set a standard for us to audit our care.

These two headings, with the five headings in the previous paragraph, should provide a useful framework to build up our audit repertoire.

How to audit

Having identified the area to audit, all the team involved in the delivery of care in this area need to devise a protocol. This means a plan consisting of the following headings:
- *Background and aims of audit.* A short introduction explaining why the particular audit was chosen and what it is hoped to achieve, along with some references if relevant to justify any expressed opinions.

Equipment needed

As well as the essential items listed in Box 37.2, a simple computer spreadsheet for presenting results graphically and a database for storing some data are useful optional extras.

Sample size for audit (rule of thumb)

How many records do I need to check to undertake this audit?

This question is often asked when practices are planning to audit groups of patients so large that it is not practical to consider checking every record. Auditing a small sample of the group may give us some idea of what is happening for an initial impression or pilot study, but if the practice wishes to have some confidence that an audit is a true measure of its performance, and not just a chance unrepresentative finding, then larger, more reliable samples will be needed. We want to choose the smallest sample that will be representative of the group to be studied and to be reasonably certain that an audit of this sample will give the same answers as an audit of the whole group.

Formulae, graphs and tables, readily available from audit sites such as the Cheshire Medical Audit Advisory Group site (see further reading below) can be used to estimate the minimum sample size needed for an audit compared with the total number in a study group (Figure 37.2).

Example

A practice wants to perform a criterion-based audit of the care of its asthma patients. There are 200 such patients on the asthma register, so, reading the graph, one can see that they will need to look at about 135 patients' records to be 95% confident that the results of the audit will be the same as if they had looked at every record.

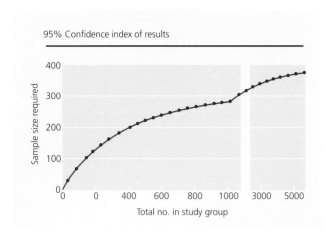

95% Confidence index of results

Figure 37.2 Graph used to calculate sample size.

The results should be expressed as percentages of the individual criteria satisfied – for example, we are 95% confident that 55–65% of our asthmatic patients have had a peak flow recorded in the past 12 months. It is important that the sample should be a random sample.

Examples of audit in primary care paediatrics

- *Structure* – We may want to look at how children's facilities are. The best judges of that are the children and their parents, so it is best to find out how we are doing from patient satisfaction survey. If worded properly, such a survey could use the parents' comments to create ideas to change the existing arrangements to be more 'child friendly'.
- *Process* – We could choose an important topic such as urinary tract infection in childhood. The sort of criteria of concern might be those shown in Box 37.3.

Box 37.3 **Possible criteria for audit of urinary tract infection care**

1 The accuracy of the diagnosis (that is, was an appropriately taken mid-stream urine specimen used to make the diagnosis, and was the result consistent with the diagnosis?).
2 Was the infection appropriately investigated and followed up?
3 Was a suitable antibiotic used?
All these criteria need to be fully discussed, justified by evidence-based published work, and then have standards applied to them. For example, the standard for taking a mid-stream urine specimen before treating a child with a suspected urinary tract infection would probably be agreed by most reasonable GPs to be 100%.

- *Outcome* – This is the most difficult subject to assess in the small populations that we deal with in general practice. However, it is possible to find a few examples. One could be to look at emergency admissions of children with asthma as a criterion of control outcome. Having sampled a group, the number of emergency admissions in a year can be measured. Having created whatever change was in mind for the children's care, the audit can be run again to see if emergency admissions have reduced.

Audit is particularly useful in primary care for assessing the effectiveness of clinics. For example, auditing various aspects of asthma care before and after instituting an asthma clinic will help ascertain whether or not the clinic is worthwhile.

Presenting audit

There is no point in doing all the hard work of audit if it is not going to make a difference to care. Take some trouble over presenting your audit. Arrange a special meeting of the primary health care team, and invite relevant local child care practitioners to attend – it is a good opportunity for networking around service collaboration. Keep records of all audits readily available in the practice meeting room and encourage students and registrars to update past audits to see how care is improving.

Further reading

As of April 2008 the National Clinical Governance Support Team closed down, with responsibility for clinical governance support, including audit, passing to strategic health authorities (SHA) in England. See your local SHA website for details of the lead advisor.

Cheshire Medical Audit Advisory Group website gives examples of formulae, graphs and tables for audit sample size: www.merseypostgradgp.nhs.uk/Vocational_Training/summ_assessment/Audit/audit_concise_guide.asp

National Audit Office *Improving Quality and Safety: Progress in Implementing Clinical Governance in Primary Care* London. National Audit Office, 2007.

National Electronic Library for Health: www.nelh.nhs.uk

NHS Quality Improvement Scotland: www.nhshealthyquality.org

Royal College of Paediatrics and Child Health audit support: www.rcpch.ac.uk/Research/CE/Guidelines/Implementation-and-Audit

CHAPTER 38

Child Abuse

Arlene Boroda

North West London NHS Trust, London, UK

OVERVIEW

- The welfare of the child is paramount.
- Effective safeguarding of children requires a multi-agency approach, following national guidance and current legislation.
- Child abuse is a spectrum of problems. Medical signs and symptoms may be the presenting problem or there may be no signs but only an allegation of abuse.
- Child abuse kills children every year. The management of child abuse requires as prompt, thorough, and careful management as for a life-threatening medical problem.
- The examination of children who may have been sexually abused should only be undertaken by specialists in the field.

Safeguarding children is everyone's responsibility. Health professionals have a key role in the recognition, investigation, and management of abuse. A high index of suspicion is essential to ensure abuse is recognized and child protection guidelines are followed to safeguard the child.

Child abuse is a culturally defined phenomenon. As Kempe (1978) wrote: 'the rights of a child to be protected from parents unable to cope at a level *assumed to be reasonable by the society in which they reside*' (Kempe, 1978, p. 263, italics added). This is a spectrum of problems. It is any intended or unintended act or omission that adversely affects a child's health, physical growth, or psychosocial development.

How big is the problem?

The true incidence of child abuse is unknown. In the UK it is estimated that each year up to 200 children are killed through child abuse; over 50% are under 1 year of age. Many more will suffer long-term consequences from physical injury and emotional damage.

Out of every 300 presentations of children to an accident and emergency department approximately 30 will have a head injury, 30 a fracture, and 5 burns or scalds resulting from accidental injury; only one child will have an injury that is non-accidental.

ABC of One to Seven, 5th edition. Edited by B. Valman. © 2010 Blackwell Publishing, ISBN: 978-1-4051-8105-1.

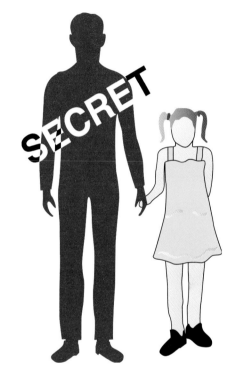

Figure 38.1 Sexual abuse is often not disclosed.

Many children do not disclose their past abuse, especially those who have been sexually abused (Figure 38.1).

Legal framework

The legal framework for child protection work is set out in the Children Act 1989, revised in 2004. Working Together to Safeguard Children (DoH 1999, revised in 2006) provides a national framework for child protection practice and guidance on interagency working.

The main principles of the Children Act 1989 are as follow:
- The welfare of the child is paramount;
- Children should be brought up within their own family whenever possible;
- Children should be safe and protected;
- Courts should avoid delay when dealing with cases involving children;
- Courts should only make an order if to do so is better than no order;

- Children should be consulted and participate in decisions about their future, they should be kept informed about what is happening to them;
- Parents continue to have responsibility even when the child is not living with them and should be kept informed and participate in decision-making about their future;

  Parents with children in need should be provided with support to care for their children.

Significant harm

The concept of significant harm, introduced in the Children Act 1989, is the threshold that should trigger when action is taken to protect the child.

Section 31 (9) of the Children Act 1989 defines 'harm' as follows:
- 'Harm' means ill-treatment or the impairment of health or development;
- 'Development' means physical, intellectual, emotional, social, or behavioural development;
- 'Health' means physical or mental health; and
- 'Ill-treatment' includes sexual abuse and forms of ill-treatment that are not physical.

When deciding if the 'harm' is significant, guidance is provided in section 31(10). Where the question of whether harm suffered by a child is significant turns on the child's health or development, his health or development shall be compared with that which could reasonably be expected of a similar child.

Recognition and management of child abuse

The recognition and management of child abuse requires a multi-disciplinary approach involving: doctors, nurses, health visitors and midwives, education, social workers, police, the child (refer to age and understanding), and the parents. An allegation of abuse made by a child can be the single most important sign of abuse.

The absence of physical signs does not exclude child abuse. Beware of unlikely or inconsistent explanations for injuries, untreated injuries, or delayed presentation for treatment (Figure 38.2). The child shows obvious signs of abuse, neglect, or failure to thrive. Numerous presentations with minor problems may be a cry for help. Always ask about previous admissions and attendances to other health professionals. Check other attendances and presentations of the same child in different departments of the same hospital or other hospitals. Consider talking to the child alone.

Professionals should record all medical findings, actions, and discussions in the notes. Information should be accessible and confidential, shared on a need-to-know basis. The case should be discussed with the clinician's supervisor and the child protection lead for the department. If possible, consult a named or designated professional for safeguarding children.

Making a referral to statutory agencies

If someone is worried that a child has been abused, a call or referral, as in the case of a professional, should be made to social care.

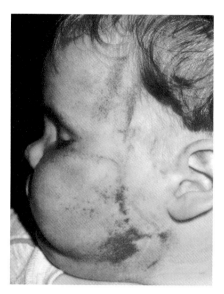

Figure 38.2 Beware of unlikely explanation for injuries (finger mark bruises).

The police should also be contacted if there are concerns that a crime has been committed. The parents and child (if the child is old enough to understand) should be told of the concern, unless it is considered that such a discussion would place the child at further risk of harm, as in sexual abuse or fabricated or induced illness by a carer. A telephone conversation should be followed by a written referral within 48 hours.

The paediatric assessment

Assessments should be holistic, well planned, and consider the emotional and physical well-being of the child. Delays should be kept to a minimum. Children should not be examined against their wishes. The consultant will decide which doctor will examine the child, depending on the level of skill and training of the clinician. Children have the right to have a same sex chaperone present. Consent must be obtained.

Do not force child to give information – ask open-ended questions. Be sympathetic to both child and parent. Careful consideration needs to be given to what questions are asked if the child has not been interviewed. Questions would be limited to specific medically related issues (write replies verbatim). The history should be taken once by the examining paediatrician and should include child's general health and development and information about the incident.

Examination should include growth parameters, vital signs, and current development. The examination is performed from top-to-toe. The genitalia are examined if the issues are a genital symptom, there is serious abuse such as multiple fractures or a severe head injury, or if child has been missing. Injuries should be recorded on a body map.

Always record the views of the child. Assess and support the emotional well-being of the child and carers. Assess and treat injuries. Photographs should be taken of injuries (Figure 38.2). Assessment is comprehensive including the presentation of the child, the general appearance, and clothing.

Feedback and discuss with the social care worker or police your findings and agree and record an action plan to safeguard the child and ensure any health needs are met.

Forensic investigation

Specific samples or tests may be needed to assist the investigation of possible child abuse, especially in acute cases. The clinician should be able to contact a paediatrician with forensic expertise or a forensic examiner from the police may assist. Samples of blood, urine, and hair may be needed for analysis for toxins under the chain of evidence procedures. Skeletal surveys and magnetic resonance imaging of the brain may detect occult injuries, especially in pre-verbal children under 2 years of age.

Admission of children to hospital

A child may need to be admitted for medical reasons such as observation of clinical signs or for tests, for further observation of parent–child interaction, or for a second medical opinion. If the parents refuse this or are uncooperative, police protection can be invoked or the Family Law Courts may assist with the issuing of orders such as Emergency Protection Orders or Interim Care Orders.

Sexual abuse

Sexual abuse is widespread and often goes unrecognized. In adults, 2–17% of women and 5–8% of men report being the victims of sexual abuse during childhood. Sexual abuse is associated with significant long-term adverse effects including depression, anxiety, and low self-esteem, sexual and relationship problems, and substance abuse.

Sexual abuse may present in a number of ways. The most common presentation is for a child or young person to make a disclosure to a trusted adult or friend. Sexually explicit behaviour, precocious sexual knowledge, excessive masturbation, anorexia, regressive behaviour, truancy, or antisocial behaviour may be indicators of sexual abuse and should lead to further enquiry. Children may present with vulvitis, vaginal bleeding or discharge, enuresis, or encopresis.

Physical signs that should arouse suspicion are as follow:
- Pregnancy, especially if the identity of the father is withheld;
- Sexually transmitted diseases;
- Bruising, abrasions of the genitalia and perianal area;
- Lacerations of the labia or posterior fourchette;
- Lacerations of the hymen and/or vaginal wall;
- Vaginal discharge or foreign body;
- Venous congestion of the anal margin;
- Anal bleeding or multiple fissures;
- Anal gaping or loss of anal sphincter tone;
- Penile injury.

Examination of children and young people who have, or may have been, sexually abused should only be undertaken by specialists in the field, with a forensic medical examiner present if the alleged incident occurred within 72 hours of presentation. The Royal College of Paediatrics and Child Health and the Faculty of Forensic and Legal Medicine have published guidance for these examinations. The use of photo-documentation, including still photographs and videos of the genital examination, assist with the follow-up of the genital medical signs. The photographs may be used for obtaining expert review of the medical findings without the need for repeat examination of the child and allow for evidence-based audit and research.

Multiple examinations, which may be distressing and abusive, should be avoided. Do not change the clothes or wash any child thought to have been sexually abused within the previous 72 hours as this may destroy forensic evidence.

In the majority of cases of sexual abuse there will be no physical findings on examination. In cases of alleged or possible assault within the last 72 hours, samples should be taken for retrieval of DNA to identify the perpetrator. Swabs may be taken from the external and internal genitalia and the rest of the body depending on the history and clinical findings.

Child death overview panels

Child death overview panels (CDOP) have been set up to review deaths of children, including the sudden infant deaths, expected and unexpected deaths. The regulatory framework in the UK is outlined in Chapter 7 of the government guidance *Working Together to Safeguard Children* (2006). Their purpose is to assess whether the index case may be one of child abuse, to safeguard the siblings in the home, and to look at trends of causes of death as part of public health initiatives, such as road safety issues, maternal and infant health, and environmental factors.

Further reading

Working Together to Safeguard Children: A Guide to Interagency Working to Safeguard and Promote the Welfare of Children. HM Government, London TSO, 2006.

Her Majesty's Stationery Office. *The Victoria Climbie Inquiry. Report of an Inquiry by Lord Lamming.* The Stationery Office, 2003.

Royal College of Paediatrics and Child Health (RCPCH) Faculty of Forensic and Legal Medicine. *Forensic Examinations in Relation to Possible Child Sexual Abuse.* RCPCH, 2007.

CHAPTER 39

Services for Children: Children's Social Care

Ron Lock

Independent Child Protection Consultant, Salisbury, UK

OVERVIEW

- A doctor has a responsibility to refer concerns about the welfare of children.
- The appropriate process is described for making these referrals.
- There is a distinction between a 'child in need' and 'a child in need of protection'.
- How social workers will respond to the doctor's referral of concerns is outlined.
- There is a spectrum of possible outcomes from child protection referrals to Children's Social Care.

In response to the Children Act 2004, the term 'Social Services Department' as a title for the local authority services delivered to children in need or for children at risk has ceased to exist, and has been replaced by a variety of different titles, although the term 'Children's Social Care' can be used generically.

The responsibility to refer concerns

It is now enshrined in the Children Act 2004 that all health professionals, among a wide variety of other agencies, must ensure that 'their functions are discharged having regard to the need to safeguard and promote the welfare of children' (Section 11), which in essence means that doctors have a statutory responsibility to address any concerns they may have about the welfare of children. Furthermore, government guidance identifies that all health professionals working with children should ensure that safeguarding and promoting their welfare forms an integral part of all stages of the care they offer. In the course of their work doctors will identify children whom they consider are in need of additional services from Children's Social Care, or who may be at risk and need protective interventions (Figure 39.1). Within the latter circumstances, it will be essential to share these concerns with the local Children's Social Care department and to make a formal referral for their advice or intervention.

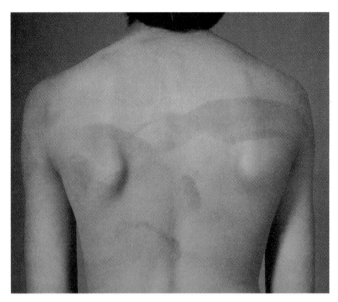

Figure 39.1 Strap mark bruises.

When judging how to respond to any concern raised regarding the welfare of a child, Children's Social Care departments work within the parameters of the Children Act 1989, which in effect means that they will need to make a judgement whether the concerns raised relate to a 'child in need' as defined in Section 17 of the Act, or that the child is suffering, or is likely to suffer significant harm, as defined in Section 47 of the same Act. The terms 'Section 17' and 'Section 47' are used as shorthand by social workers to refer to these different levels of concern.

A child in need

The term 'child in need' defines children who are vulnerable and are unlikely to reach or maintain a satisfactory level of health and development, or that their health and development will be significantly impaired, unless services are provided to address these issues. This would also relate to disabled children. The key question is what would be likely happen to this child if services from Children's Social Care are not provided.

ABC of One to Seven, 5th edition. Edited by B. Valman. © 2010 Blackwell Publishing, ISBN: 978-1-4051-8105-1.

A child in need of protection

The concept of 'significant harm' was introduced within the Children Act 1989, in that if it is considered that a child is already suffering, or is likely to suffer, significant harm, then such a level of concern justifies a compulsory level of intervention by Children's Social Care. This will relate to those circumstances where there is concern about physical, sexual, or emotional abuse, or of neglect of the child. The local Safeguarding Children Procedures gives the formal definitions of each type of abuse.

Thresholds and eligibility criteria

Each Children's Social Care department will likely have a published set of eligibility criteria, which will determine the priority they will give to certain levels of concern or child need, and the speed with which they will respond to a referral. While those concerns in relation to serious child abuse allegations will require a formal child protection enquiry to take place within 24 hours, other less serious concerns will be afforded a lower priority for service as detailed in their eligibility criteria. For example, in respect of referrals that relate to a 'child in need', then the priority afforded to the response may make a distinction between those children who are likely to be considerably impaired if the support services are not provided, rather than those deemed unlikely to achieve a reasonable standard of health or development without them. Each Children's Social Care department will have different levels of eligibility criteria dependent upon local issues.

It is important that if a health professional refers a child for whom there is concern regarding allegations of child abuse, or is in the health professional's opinion subject to significant harm, then the first contact with Children's Social Care should be prefaced with the statement that the individual 'wishes to make a child protection referral', which would then make it clear which level of concern is to be addressed.

First steps

Ideally, and if time allows, the health professional should initially discuss concerns with the 'named' or designated health professional for safeguarding children, within the relevant NHS Trust or Primary Care Trust. The named professional (e.g. nurse, GP, or paediatrician) has a key role in providing advice and expertise to fellow professionals on the subject of safeguarding children.

Many Children's Social Care departments, as part of local interagency arrangements, require the completion of a referral form in order to give the necessary information about the child and the concerns. While the completion of the form is likely to be the first step where it is considered the child is 'in need', if a child protection referral is made, then the process should not be delayed, and a telephone call immediately made, with the completed referral form acting as confirmation of concern.

The referral

In order for the referral to be accepted and responded to effectively, it is important that the essential information is conveyed to Children's Social Care. Apart from the child's basic details, clear evidence and examples of reasons for concern should be given, as well as the doctor's professional opinion, based upon that evidence and other observations. The medical view of the child's circumstances, condition, or injuries will be of particular importance and relevance to the social worker.

When making the referral, discussion with Children's Social Care should include an agreement regarding what the parents and child will be told, by whom and when. This will help in future contact with the child and family.

Ensure that any telephone referral is followed up by letter (or via the locally agreed referral form) within 48 hours. It is a requirement that Children's Social Care then acknowledge written referral in writing, within 24 hours of its receipt. If this has not been received within 3 working days, it is important to follow up with Children's Social Care.

Information sharing

If there is concern that a child may be suffering significant harm, then the child's safety must be the overriding consideration when making a decision to share information about them. While generally, consent should be sought from the parents regarding sharing information or when making a referral, in exceptional circumstances it may increase risk to try to seek their permission or agreement. Even if they do not consent, you may need to override this based on the circumstances of the case, and of the risk to the child.

Talking with children and parents or carers

In addition to having prior discussion with the parents, it is advised good practice to discuss concerns with the child also, as appropriate to their age and understanding, and to seek their agreement to making any referral. Clearly, this is much less likely with the younger child, and although it may nevertheless be appropriate to talk to a young child about the presenting concerns, clearly their agreement would not be necessary. It is important to be aware that a serious child protection concern may lead to a criminal investigation, and therefore it would not be appropriate to ask leading questions of a child or attempt to investigate the concerns. The health professional's role is to identify the concerns clearly and then to refer the matter to Children's Social Care for them to decide how to respond.

Response to concerns by social workers

The Children's Social Care social worker will need to decide within 1 working day what action to take in respect of the referral, and they should inform the health professional accordingly.

The first action by a social worker on receipt of the referral should be to undertake an initial assessment which needs to be completed within 7 working days. This is a brief assessment to determine if the child is in need, the nature of any services required, from where and within what timescales, and whether a more detailed assessment is required. The initial assessment needs to include the collation of information from the family and other professionals regarding the child's needs, and the child should be seen and, where appropriate, spoken to by the social worker as part of the process.

Based on the findings from the initial assessment, a decision will be made by Children's Social Care regarding what action, if any, the social workers will take. It could mean that they decide to refer the child and family for support from another agency.

A decision could be made to undertake a core assessment if it becomes apparent that the concerns presented are such that a more in-depth and detailed analysis of the child's circumstances is required. A core assessment must be undertaken within 35 working days, and while the social worker will take the lead on this, each professional involved with the child and family will be asked for their information and opinion on the child's developmental needs, the parents' or carers' capacity to respond appropriately to those needs, and the wider family and environmental factors. The outcome of the core assessment should identify a clear way forward for addressing the child's needs.

If the referral relates to a serious child protection concern, then although the above processes may be initiated, it is more likely that a strategy discussion will take place between the social work manager and a police manager, to decide on the need and type of intervention required. A health professional's input may be requested as part of that strategy discussion. A possible outcome is that a child protection enquiry is immediately conducted (often referred to as a Section 47 Investigation/Enquiry) and the child's circumstances and levels of risk formally investigated as a matter of urgency. A child protection medical is likely to be required, usually conducted

by a consultant paediatrician. If the concerns are very serious then an emergency protection order for a period up to 8 days could be sought via the courts by the social worker.

Commitment to continuous interagency collaboration

It is important to be aware that the part of the health professional in the process of safeguarding children does not end at the point of referral. If it has been identified that the child has been suffering significant harm or is likely to, then there would be child protection conferences to contribute to, as well as to any subsequent child protection plan.

Further reading

Beckett C. *Child Protection: An Introduction.* Sage Publications, London, 2003.

Department for Education and Skills (DfES). *Information Sharing: Practitioner's Guide: Integrated Working to Improve Outcomes for Children and Young People.* DfES Publications, 2006.

Department for Education and Skills (DfES). *What to Do If You Are Worried That a Child Is Being Abused.* DfES Publications, 2006.

Department of Health, Home Office, Department for Education and Employment. *Working Together to Safeguard Children: A Guide to Interagency Working to Safeguard and Promote the Welfare of Children.* HM Government, London, 2006.

Munro E. *Effective Child Protection.* Sage Publications, London, 2002.

CHAPTER 40

Useful Information

Bernard Valman

Northwick Park Hospital and Imperial College London, UK

Acute herpetic gingivostomatitis

Primary infection of the mucous membranes of the mouth is the most common infection with herpes simplex in childhood. It usually occurs at 1–4 years. A high fever and refusal to eat are accompanied by red swollen gums which bleed easily. There are white plaques about 3 mm in diameter or painful shallow ulcers with a red rim on the buccal mucosa, gums, tongue, and palate, and the regional lymph nodes are enlarged and tender (Figure 40.1). This is a self-limiting disease which resolves in about 10 days.

Treatment consists of keeping the mouth clean and maintaining hydration. Children who are seen within 3 days of the onset of severe symptoms can be given a course of oral or intravenous aciclovir. This treatment is less likely to be effective if given later in the illness. The child might have to be admitted to hospital to prevent dehydration from refusal to drink. Regular doses of paracetamol elixir and frequent small volumes of a glucose solution or milk should be given. Paracetamol suppositories can be given to children who refuse all oral fluids. Drinks and solids should be offered when oral or rectal paracetamol has the maximum effect, which is 30 minutes to 4 hours after the dose has been given. Fluids may cause less pain if a drinking straw is used, and jelly and ice cream may be taken easily, but citrus juices should be avoided because they increase the pain.

Cervical lymphadenopathy (non-suppurative)

In children aged over 2 years cervical lymphadenopathy usually affects the tonsillar nodes, but more distal nodes in the neck may be affected (Figure 40.2). Viral or bacterial infection in the upper respiratory tract spreads to these lymph nodes, which change in size with each acute infection. Despite these wide changes in size the nodes seldom disappear completely for several years.

If the nodes do not change in size between two observations 1 month apart the possibility of tuberculosis should be considered and a tuberculin test performed.

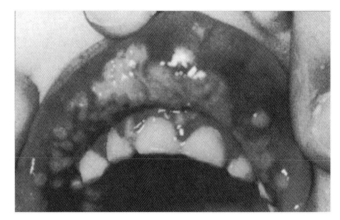

Figure 40.1 Acute herpetic gingivostomatitis.

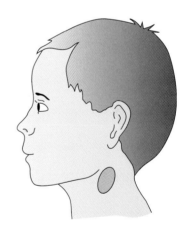

Figure 40.2 Cervical lymphadenopathy.

Generalized lymphadenopathy suggests the possibility of infectious mononucleosis, leukaemia, or lymphoma. A full blood count should be performed and a blood film examined for evidence of leukaemia. If the Monospot screening test for infectious mononucleosis is negative blood should be taken for toxoplasma and cytomegalovirus antibody titres and bone marrow examination should be considered. If all these tests are negative a surgeon should be consulted to consider biopsy to exclude malignant disease.

ABC of One to Seven, 5th edition. Edited by B. Valman. © 2010 Blackwell Publishing, ISBN: 978-1-4051-8105-1.

Anal fissure

An anal fissure causes severe pain on defecation because the lesion is stretched as the stool is being passed. Fresh blood may be seen on the surface of the stool. The mucosal tear, which may occur at any point on the circumference of the mucocutaneous junction of the anus, may be visible but the lesion may be very small or too high to be seen. Fissures are usually the result of trauma to the anal margin by the passage of hard stools. This constipation may be the result of inadequate intake of fluid during a febrile illness. As a result of the pain the child resists defecation and the stools become hard and the symptoms more severe. Without treatment chronic constipation sometimes occurs with overflow diarrhoea.

The stools are kept soft by ensuring an adequate fluid intake and the addition of polyethylene glycol (Movicol) for 8 weeks. The child then regains confidence that defecation will not be painful. It is essential that this course of treatment should be completed, as a fissure takes a long time to heal. Surgical excision of the fissure or stretching of the anus is rarely needed if medical treatment is adequate.

A rectal polyp is a rarer cause of rectal bleeding, but the absence of pain helps to distinguish it from a fissure.

Constipation

Constipation is an alteration in bowel habit with the passage of hard stools and a reduction in the frequency of stools. Normal children may pass stools between four times a day and once every 2 days, but the stool is soft and the width of the stool is appropriate for a child of that age. The width of the stool reflects the width of the colon (Figure 40.3) Any child with an acute illness tends to eat and drink less than normal and passes fewer stools. Apart from ensuring that fluid intake is adequate no treatment is required. If there is an inadequate intake of fluid the stools may become hard and produce an anal fissure. The pain produced during defecation by the fissure may make children reluctant to pass stools so that they hold them back by crossing their legs. Several days may pass before the child passes a formed stool, which is then voluminous and may cause severe pain.

Colonic inertia with overflow soiling

If the child persists in refusing to pass stools chronic constipation follows. The whole colon becomes distended with firm stool and the reflex urge to defecate is lost as a result of the persistent distension of the rectum (Figure 40.4). At this stage enormous masses of faeces may be palpated through the abdominal wall and detected on

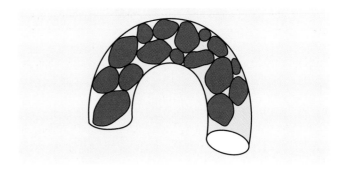

Figure 40.4 Secondary megacolon.

rectal examination. Liquid stool may trickle continuously around the masses and escape with gas through the anus. Parents may complain about this continual loss of fluid stool and call it diarrhoea without realising that there is underlying constipation. In some children there is no obvious history of an anal fissure but bowel training has been attempted before the age of 2 years.

By the time the child is seen by a doctor the problem has often been present for several months or years and any emotional problems present may be primary or secondary to the physical problem. Most of these children can be managed by medicines, and a child psychiatrist should be consulted about those who do not improve quickly or who relapse.

The cause of the problem is discussed with both parents and the child using simple diagrams, and they should be told that aperients will be needed for a prolonged period, at least for a year, otherwise relapse will occur. The following drugs are given initially together:

1 Senna extract (Senokot) 5 mL at night; the dose of senna extract is increased by 5 mL every third night until there is a daily bowel action or until the maximum dose of 20 mL is given; and
2 Polyethylene glycol (Movicol).

Senna acts by propelling the stool and polyethylene glycol by softening it. The child should be asked to sit on the lavatory at the same time each day to encourage reflex defecation, and must be seen initially each week and then at monthly intervals to ensure that the medicine is being taken. When there has been a daily bowel action for 1 month the doses of the drugs are reduced gradually over the subsequent 3 months. Relapse is common and the parents should be warned about this possibility. Suppositories, enemas, and manual removal of faeces can rarely be justified except in children with cerebral palsy.

Passing stools in unusual places such as behind curtains indicates a severe behaviour disorder, which needs referral to a child psychiatrist.

Iron deficiency anaemia

In children less than 2 years of age iron deficiency is common. The prevalence may be as high as 50% in some populations. Rapid growth and low content of iron in milk causes the high prevalence of iron deficiency. Preterm infants are born with low iron stores. Iron deficiency anaemia can be prevented by giving supplementary iron to preterm infants and by starting solids containing iron no

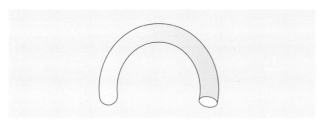

Figure 40.3 Normal colon.

later than the age of 6 months. Chronic microscopic bleeding may occur in some infants who have received whole cow's milk. Iron deficiency may have a detrimental effect on behaviour or intellectual function which may be reversible with iron therapy and changes in diet. Pallor, tiredness, irritability, and anorexia may occur. Anaemia may be suspected by the colour of the tongue or conjunctivae but a clinical diagnosis alone is unreliable.

There are two approaches to the management of suspected iron deficiency anaemia. If a full blood count shows microcytic anaemia (low mean cell volume) iron supplements are given for a month. The full blood count is repeated with estimations of plasma ferritin and haemoglobin electrophoresis. If the haemoglobin level has not increased there is a possibility of non-compliance, thalassaemia trait, or lead poisoning and a blood lead level should be considered.

An alternative approach is to perform a full blood count, plasma ferritin level, and haemoglobin electrophoresis at the first visit. If the plasma ferritin is low, which indicates low stores of iron, iron supplements should be given for a month. Repeat full blood count, ferritin level, and haemoglobin electrophoresis are performed. If there is no improvement in the haemoglobin level, a blood lead level is considered. In the presence of iron deficiency, thalassaemia trait may be masked and the haemoglobin electrophoresis should be repeated when the serum ferritin level has become normal (see below).

Investigations for a cause of bleeding should be carried out if the cause of anaemia is not detected by the above investigations, the anaemia fails to respond to iron therapy, or recurs.

Iron supplements are given for 2–3 months to replete the iron stores. The consumption of milk is limited to 450 mL per day to encourage the consumption of more solids containing iron. Dietary sources of iron include red meat and poultry, dark green vegetables, pulses, bread, and chapatti. Iron absorption from food is increased when eaten in combination with a food rich in vitamin C – for example, fruit or vegetables.

Haemoglobinopathies: normal haematological values and diagnosis

Normal ranges for haemoglobin concentrations and red cell counts vary with age (Table 40.1). The normal ranges printed on standard report forms should be age related.

The child with severe anaemia caused by sickle cell anaemia or thalassaemia major receives an abnormal gene from each parent,

who has no symptoms. In sickle cell anaemia there is a chronic haemolytic anaemia with superimposed crises due to local sickling, marrow aplasia, or acute haemolysis. Hypoxaemia causes deformity of the red cells with local sickling, which results in blocking of capillaries and further hypoxia and sickling (Figure 40.5). Ischaemia distal to the local sickling lesion causes bone, chest, or abdominal pain or infarcts in the brain, spleen, or kidneys. The child's parents who both have the trait (or a child with the trait) develop a sickling crisis or mild anaemia only if very severe prolonged hypoxaemia occurs. Diagnosis depends on detecting haemoglobin S alone on the haemoglobin electrophoresis of the child with sickle cell anaemia and haemoglobin S and haemoglobin A in both parents.

The most common type of thalassaemia in the UK is β thalassaemia, in which there is reduced synthesis of the β chain of globin leading to reduced synthesis of haemoglobin A and hypochromic microcytic anaemia. Synthesis of haemoglobin F and haemoglobin A2 are not affected and so the percentages of haemoglobin F and A2 are increased.

Two genes for thalassaemia are present in children with thalassaemia major and one in those with thalassaemia trait. Children with thalassaemia major usually need regular blood transfusions and desferrioxamine throughout their life. If blood transfusion is inadequate they have severe chronic haemolytic anaemia with a very large liver and spleen and later enlargement of the frontal and malar bones due to bone marrow hyperplasia. Thalassaemia trait causes mild or no anaemia. The blood picture is similar to that of iron deficiency anaemia but the mean cell volume is disproportionately reduced compared with the red cell count and haemoglobin levels; the MCV : RBC ratio is less than 12 and the serum ferritin is normal. The diagnosis is confirmed by finding a raised percentage

Table 40.1 Normal ranges for haemoglobin.

Age	Haemoglobin (g/L)	Mean corpuscular volume (fL)
½–1 year	105–135	70–80
1–4 years	110–140	70–82
4–7 years	115–135	76–86
Adult	130–150	80–100

Mean corpuscular haemoglobin concentration is constant throughout life (300–340 g/L).

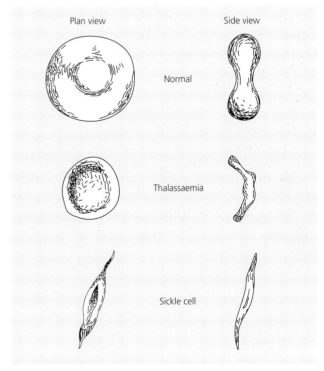

Figure 40.5 Shapes of cells in haemoglobinopathies.

of haemoglobin A2 or haemoglobin F, or both. A child may have both iron deficiency and thalassaemia trait. A 2-month course of supplementary oral iron and repeat full blood count, plasma ferritin level, and haemoglobin electrophoresis will clarify the problem.

If thalassaemia trait or sickle cell trait is suspected during a routine antenatal clinic blood count, the father should also be tested immediately. If he has a similar abnormality the possibility that the fetus has a severe haemoglobinopathy should be considered and further expert opinion sought as a matter of urgency.

Rickets

Inadequate bone mineralization causes rickets which is most commonly caused by deficiency of vitamin D. Bowing and distortion of bones and muscle weakness are the main features. The amount of vitamin D required in infancy is related to the stores built up *in utero* and subsequent exposure to sunlight. Breastfed babies, particularly preterm or born to vitamin D deficient mothers may become deficient. Most formula milks and supplementary feeds contain adequate vitamin D to prevent deficiency. Poor mineralization in the newborn and young children may also be caused by inadequate intake of phosphate or calcium during long-term parenteral nutrition.

Vitamin D deficiency can be prevented if babies who are breastfed after the age of 6 months and all infants receiving less than 0.5 L (1 pint) of formula milk (which contains added vitamins) per day receive supplementary drops of vitamins A, C, and D until the age of 4 years. All preterm infants receive supplementary vitamin D.

The diagnosis is confirmed by measuring the plasma calcium, phosphate, alkaline phosphatase, and vitamin D levels and a radiograph of a wrist should be considered. Vitamin D levels are lowest towards the end of winter and highest in the summer because of the effects of sunlight. Rickets brought about by nutritional deficiency is treated with vitamin D. Children receiving pharmacological doses of vitamin D should have the blood concentration of calcium checked at weekly intervals initially to avoid hypercalcaemia.

Jaundice caused by hepatitis

Infectious hepatitis is most commonly caused by hepatitis A virus. Before jaundice appears there is often headache, anorexia, nausea, vomiting, abdominal pain, and occasionally fever. The liver may be enlarged and tender, and the spleen and lymph nodes may also be enlarged. Jaundice starts as the fever subsides, and as the jaundice increases the child's appetite improves. The urine is dark because of bile and the stools may be very pale. Jaundice lasts for 8–11 days. In children under 3 years, especially those in institutions, hepatitis may occur without jaundice.

If children want to stay in bed they should be allowed to, but prolonged bed rest is not essential. While there is anorexia or vomiting small volumes of glucose–electrolyte mixture flavoured with fruit juice should be given every hour during the day. As the appetite returns a normal diet may be given with no restriction of fat. No drugs are needed although some clinicians recommend vitamin supplements. Viral hepatitis is one of the mildest childhood infections and the prognosis is excellent.

The patient is potentially infectious for no more than a week after the onset of jaundice. The virus is spread by the faecal–oral route, and spread can be prevented by handwashing and by boiling food utensils for at least a minute.

When features are typical no tests are needed and the children should be nursed in their own home. Drowsiness or jaundice lasting longer than 2 weeks should prompt a further opinion.

Prophylaxis – Hepatitis A vaccine is the preferred method to prevent secondary cases in close contacts of a confirmed case of hepatitis A, within 7 days of onset of the disease in the primary case.

Type A viral hepatitis has an average incubation period of 30 days (range 15–40 days). Most human sera, and therefore human globulin preparations, contain antibody, and if this is given by injection during the incubation period it protects against the disease. The indications for giving this injection are controversial and vary between countries and units. Hepatitis A infections in children are usually mild and confer lifelong immunity, but the incidence of such infections has declined recently in northern Europe, although in southern Europe most people are infected by the time they are adults. In adults hepatitis A is more severe but rarely causes persisting or serious liver disease. In future it is more likely that adults will contract the disease from their children. Nevertheless, globulin should be used only within the incubation period, and preferably within 15 days of contact, and if there is some special reason to fear hepatitis in a sibling or adult.

In countries outside the UK, where hepatitis B is common, different advice on prophylaxis may be more appropriate.

Vulvovaginitis

Vulvovaginitis may cause dysuria, vulval irritation, or a yellow stain on the pants, but the only abnormality to be seen may be a thin, yellowish-grey, vaginal discharge. The symptoms and even the results of a urine examination may be wrongly attributed to a urinary infection. Swabs (moistened with 0.9% sodium chloride solution) of the secretions are sent to the laboratory for microscopy and culture and the mother is taught how to collect a specimen for threadworm ova. When the child wakes in the morning, ova can be collected from the perianal skin with a moist swab.

The only infections indicating specific antimicrobial treatment are those caused by group A streptococci, gonococci, *Monilia*, or *Trichomonas* (Box 40.1). Antibiotic treatment of infection with other organisms may result in fungal overgrowth causing iatrogenic disease. If no pathogens are detected the symptoms may be a result of poor perineal hygiene and may resolve after twice daily baths. Detergents in poorly rinsed pants or 'bubble baths' may

---

Box 40.1 **Causes of vulvovaginitis**

- Pathogens
- Poor perineal hygiene
- Insufficiently rinsed pants
- Bubble baths
- Thin vaginal mucosa
- Foreign body

cause a chemical vulvovaginitis. The symptoms in remaining girls are usually related to a thin, unstimulated, vaginal mucosa. If the problem needs more than reassurance, the child should be referred to a gynaecologist who may prescibe a mild oestrogen cream for 2 weeks. This tiny dose thickens the mucosa. Longer treatment may cause withdrawal bleeding. A profuse, purulent, blood-streaked, offensive discharge or symptoms that recur despite these measures are indications for referral to a gynaecologist to exclude a foreign body in the vagina.

Some useful drugs

Children treated at home and most of those in hospital need oral drugs three times a day. They should be given before meals and the child need not be woken specially for the drug. Some preparations, particularly the penicillins, have an unpleasant taste and the medicine should not be mixed with food as the child may then hate both. Syrup, which is a sucrose solution that forms the base of most elixirs, may cause dental caries if it is given regularly for a long time. Some liquid preparations have no sugar. The concentration of the drug in the elixir should be high to provide a minimum volume. In difficult 1 to 3-year-olds wrapping the child securely in a blanket may prevent spillage if only one adult is present to give the medicine. If a child will not accept a drug on a spoon the drug can be measured in a medicine syringe or a disposable syringe (with no needle) and squirted on to the child's tongue. The doses given here are suitable for children aged 1–7 years.

Amoxycillin oral 125–250 mg 3 times daily
Ampicillin oral 125–250 mg 4 times daily
  iv 25–50 mg/kg (max 1 g) every 6 hours
Benzylpenicillin im or iv 25–50 mg/kg every 4–6 hours
Carbamazepine oral 5–20 mg/kg/24 hours. Start with small dose
Cefotaxime iv 50 mg/kg every 8–12 hours
Ceftazidime iv or im 25–50 mg/kg every 8 hours
Cefalexin oral 125 mg 3 times daily
Chloral hydrate oral 30 mg/kg at night
Chlorpheniramine oral 1 mg 3 times daily
  im, iv 2.5–5 mg. Repeat if required
Diazepam iv 300–400 microgram/kg slowly
Diazepam rectal solution (Stesolid) 5–10 mg. Repeated after 10 minutes if necessary
Erythromycin oral 250 mg 4 times daily
Flucloxacillin oral 125–250 mg 4 times daily
  iv 50 mg/kg 4 times daily
Gentamicin iv 2.5 mg/kg 3 times daily
Hydrocortisone iv 2–4 mg/kg per dose
Naloxone im or iv 10 microgram/kg per dose. Can be repeated after 3 minutes
Nitrofurantoin oral 1 mg/kg single dose daily as maintenance dose
Nystatin oral 100,000 units 4 times daily after food
Paracetamol oral 120–250 mg every 4–6 hours (maximum of 4 doses in 24 hours)
Phenobarbital oral 1–1.5 mg/kg twice daily initially
Phenoxymethyl penicillin oral 125 mg 4 times daily
Phenytoin oral 1.5–2.5 mg/kg twice daily initially
Sodium ironedetate oral 2.5 mL 3 times daily
Sodium valproate oral 5–7.5 mg/kg twice daily initially
Trimethoprim oral 4 mg/kg twice daily

Toys

Toys appropriate for a child's development are useful in assessment but are also necessary to ensure that the child cooperates during the examination (Figure 40.6). Suitable toys for various ages include: press-up animals, elasticated collapse–return toys, snowstorms or shaking and turning toys, kaleidoscopes, miniature people, cars, crayons, telephones, rag dolls, crayons and paper, dolls' houses and dolls' furniture, wooden puzzles, fitting plastic beakers, and plastic rings on a pole. Suitable books include Ladybird first picture books 1–3 years and Mister Men 3–6 years. A glove puppet is also very useful for shy children, who will sometimes talk to a puppet but not to an adult. It can also be used to divert attention.

Guidance for parents of children with various illnesses or disabilities

The Contact a Family directory. Tel: 0808 808 3555 (www.cafamily. org.uk). This charity provides advice, information, and support to parents of all disabled children and enables parents to get in touch with other families with a similar condition.

Asthma
The Chest, Heart & Stroke Association. Tel: 020 7566 0300. Fax: 020 7490 2686.

Blindness
Royal National Institute of Blind People (RNIB), 105 Judd Street, London WC1H 9NE. Tel: 08457 669 999. Fax: 020 7388 2034. www.helpline@rnib.org.uk

Cerebral palsy and spasticity
SCOPE, 6 Market Road, London N7 9PW. Tel: 0808 800 3333. www.scope.org.uk/response

Coeliac disease
Coeliac Society, PO Box 220, High Wycombe, Bucks HP11 2HY. Tel: 01494 437 278. www.24dr.com/reference/contact/group/coeliac_

Crying
BM Cry-sis, London WC1N 3XX. Tel: 08451 228 669. www.cry-sis. org.uk. For parents of babies who cry excessively.

Cystic fibrosis
Cystic Fibrosis Trust. Tel: 0845 859 1000.

Deafness
National Deaf Children's Society, 16 Dufferin Street, London EC1Y 8UR. Tel: 020 7490 8656.

Royal National Institute for the Deaf, 19 Featherstone Street, London EC1Y 8SL. Tel: 0870 605 0123. www.informationline@ rnid.org

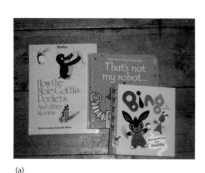

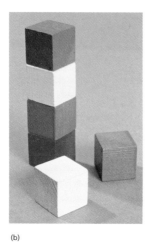

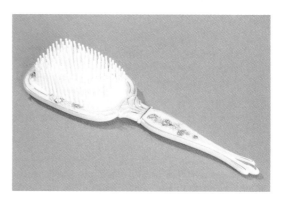

(a)

(b)

(c)

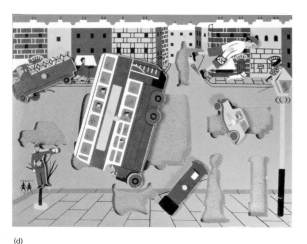

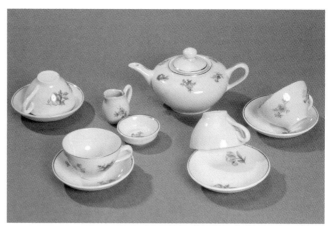

(d)

(e)

Figure 40.6 Appropriate toys: (a) books; (b) small bricks; (c) hairbrush; (d) puzzle; (e) miniature tea set.

Diabetes
The British Diabetic Association is known as Diabetes UK, Macleod House, 10 Parkway, London NW1 7AA. Tel: 020 7424 1000. Fax: 020 7424 1001. www.info@diabetes.org.uk

Disablement
Disabled Living Foundation, 380–384 Harrow Road, London W9 2HU. Tel: 0845 130 9177. www.advice@dlf.org.uk

Down's syndrome
Down's Syndrome Association, Langdon Down Centre, 2a Langdon Park, Teddington TW11 9PS. Tel: 0845 230 0372. Fax: 0845 230 0373. www.info@downs-syndrome.org.uk

Eczema
National Eczema Society, Hill House, Highgate Hill, London N19 5NA. Tel: 0800 089 1122. Fax: 020 7281 6395. www.eczema.org

Epilepsy
British Epilepsy Association known as Epilepsy UK. Tel: 0808 800 5050. www.helpline@epilepsy.org.uk

Invalidity
Invalid children's aid nationwide. For children with communication problems. I CAN, 8 Wakley Street, London EC1V 7QE. Tel: 0845 225 4071. Fax: 0845 225 4072. www.info@ican.org.uk

Learning disability
Mencap, 123 Golden Lane, London EC1Y 0RT. Tel: 020 7454 0454. Fax: 020 7608 3254. www. help@mencap.org.uk

Acknowledgements

I thank Dr Benjamin Jacobs for his constructive review of Chapter 7 (Asthma).

I thank Susan Thomason, assisted by Máire Sullivan, of the Department of Medical Illustration at Northwick Park Hospital, who has taken several of the photographs used in this edition. A small number of photographs were reproduced from previous editions and were taken by Richard Bowlby, Joanna Fairclough, Brian Pashley, Jeanette McKenzie, and Ann Shields of the Department of Medical Illustration at Northwick Park Hospital.

The remaining illustrations were supplied as follows:

Tonsillitis and otitis media: illustration of eardrum and grommet from Valman B. *Keeping Babies and Children Healthy*. Martin Dunitz, London, 1985.

Asthma: the peak flow chart was reproduced from Godfrey S, *et al. British Journal of Diseases of the Chest* 1970; **64**: 15.

Chronic diarrhoea: jejunal biopsy histology, Professor G. Slavin.

Urinary tract infection: antibiotic sensitivity disc, courtesy of Oxoid Ltd; kidney scan, Dr Brendan Twomey.

Enuresis: the first illustration was adapted with permission from Dr M.A. Salmon and Spastic International Medical Publications from *Bladder Control and Enuresis* and the fifth by permission of Professor Roy Meadow.

Systolic murmurs: the illustrations of ventricular septal defect and patent ductus arteriosus were adapted from Hull D, Johnstone D.I. *Essential Paediatrics*. Churchill Livingstone, 1987.

Growth failure: the growth charts of 2–5 years and 0–19 years were adapted from those published by the Child Growth Foundation.

Obesity: the BMI chart is published by permission of the Child Growth Foundation.

Infectious diseases: the illustrations were adapted from Krugman S, Katz S.L. *Infectious Diseases of Children*, 7th edn. C.V. Mosby, St Louis, 1981.

Recurrent headache: CT brain scan, Dr David Katz.

Accidents: illustrations, RoSPA and Department of Transport.

For all photographs apart from those mentioned specifically above Dr H.B. Valman retains the copyright.

Index

Note: page numbers in *italics* refer to figures, those in **bold** refer to tables and boxes

abdomen
  distension 39
  radiography 33
  tenderness 98
abdominal pain 28–31
  anaphylaxis 42
  emotional factors 32, 33
  history 32
  physical disease 33
  prognosis 34
  pyelonephritis 44
  recurrent 30–31, 32–4, 132
  social factors 32, 33
  typhoid fever 67
abscess
  intracranial 84, *85*
  peritonsillar 14
absence epilepsy 80–81
abuse *see* child abuse
accidents 90–93
  see also non-accidental injury; trauma
acetylcysteine 88
achondroplasia 56
aciclovir 66, 70, 147
acid substances 87
acute assessment unit 135
adenoidectomy, indications 17
adrenaline 18, 42
aggression 106
airway
  life support 100
  obstruction 18, 94
alae nasi, flaring 11
alcohol poisoning 89
allergens
  atopic eczema 69
  avoidance 24
allergic reactions 42
ambulatory paediatrics 134–5
ampicillin, drug rash 61
anaemia
  haemolytic 66
  iron deficiency 148–9, 150
  thalassaemia 149–50
anal fissure 148
anaphylaxis 42
androgens 55

ankle hyperextension 118
antibiotics 151
  acute bronchitis 10–11
  cystic fibrosis 41
  impetigo 71
  meningitis 37–8
  otitis media 15
  pneumonia 11
  scarlet fever 66
  sensitivity testing 44, *45*
  tonsillitis 14
  typhoid fever 68
  urinary tract infection 44–5
    prophylaxis 47
  vulvovaginitis 150
  whooping cough 12, 37
anticoagulants 87
anticonvulsant drugs 78, 80, 81, 82, 97
antidepressants, poisoning 88
antihistamines 70
  poisoning 89
antisocial behaviour 106
anxiety 106
  abdominal pain 34
  maternal of toddlers 3
  separation 5
aorta, coarctation 51
aortic stenosis 51
aplastic crisis 66
apnoea, sleep 17
appendicitis 28–9, 31, 33–4
  hospital admission 135
appetite, reduction 57
appointment systems 132
arm, joint laxity 118
arthritis
  juvenile 119
  septic **104**, 119
Asperger's syndrome 108
assisted ventilation
  anaphylaxis 42
  bag and mask 95
asthma 21–2, *23*, 24–7
  acute attacks 26
  allergen avoidance 24
  assessment 22, *23*
  bronchial 11, 13, 132
  children under 2 years 27
  diagnosis 21
  drug treatment 24–6

guidance for parents 151
  hospital admission 26–7, 135
  management 24
  symptom diary 22, *23*
atopic eczema 66, 69–70, 71
atrial septal defect 51
atropine 87
attention deficit hyperactivity disorder (ADHD)
    108, 109, 113
  referral 132
  school problems 112
audiogram *16*
audit
  equipment 139
  presentation 140
  primary care 138–40
  procedure 139
  results 140
  sample size 139–40
auriscope 15
autism spectrum disorder 108, 109, 112, 113

back blows 19
bacterial infections
  gastroenteritis 36
  laryngotracheitis 19
  napkin dermatitis 72
  otitis media 14–15
  secondary 69
  tonsillitis 14, 17
  urinary tract 44
  see also named infections
bag and mask ventilation 95
barbiturates, poisoning 87–8
barrier nursing 136–7
barrier preparations 72
BCG vaccination 13
beclometasone 24, 25
beds 9
bedtime ritual 7
behaviour modification techniques, migraine 84
behaviour problems 105–7, 132, 148
  habitual behaviour 4, 105
  toddlers 4, 5
benzoic acid compound 76
beta$_2$-agonists 24, 25, 26, 27
bladder
  control 5
  distended 48
Blount's disease 116

body mass index (BMI) *58*
bone age 56
bone disease 56
bone scan 121
Bordetella pertussis (whooping cough) 11, *12*, 37
bowel control 5
breastfeeding 125
  HIV treatment 68
  neonatal unit 137
  vitamin D deficiency 150
breath-holding attacks 81, 105
breathing, life support 100–101
bronchiolitis 11, 13
  hospital admission 135
  respiratory rate 97
bronchitis 10
  acute 10–11
  recurrent 11, 13
bronchodilator drugs 26, 27
bronchopneumonia 11
budesonide 18
built environment 93
bullying 114
burns, stridor 19

calamine lotion 66
calcineurin inhibitors 70
calcium levels 150
calorie intake reduction 57, 59
Campylobacter 36
Candida 71
  HIV/AIDS 68
car seats 91
carbamazepine 80, 81, 88
cardiac compression, external 101
cardiac failure, congestive 97
cardiopulmonary resuscitation 101
care
  definition 139
  respite 110
  secondary 128
  see also primary care; social care
carers 110
  talking about social care concerns 145
carotid pulse 95
cataracts, rubella in pregnancy 67
caustic substances 87
cavernous haemangiomas 75
cerebral palsy 108, 109
  epilepsy 80
  guidance for parents 151
  limp *120*, 121
cerebral tumours 84, 121
cervical lymphadenopathy 147
charts, nocturnal enuresis 48–9
chest physiotherapy, whooping cough 12
chest radiograph
  asthma 22
  respiratory infections 11, 12
  tuberculosis 13
  whooping cough 37
chest thrusts 19
chickenpox 65–6, 137
  vesicles 61, *62*
child abuse 113, 141–3
  assessment 142–3
  forensic investigation 143

hospital admission 143
  legal framework 141–2, 143
  management 142
  photographs 142, 143
  recognition 142
  referral 142
  see also non-accidental injury
Child and Adult Mental Health Service
    (CAMHS) 109, 112, 113
child death overview panels (CDOP) 143
child development 125, **126**
  services 109
child health services 128
  day-care 132–3
  outpatient clinics 131–2
child health surveillance 123, 125, 128, **129**
child in need 144
child protection 130, 141–2
  child in need 145
  referral 146
Children Act (1989, 2004) 141–2, 144
children's centres 124
Children's Social Care departments 144, 145
  decision making 146
  referral 5
Chinese herbal medicine, atopic eczema 69
chloral hydrate 7
choking 19
chronic fatigue syndrome 106–7
  infectious mononucleosis 67
circulation, life support 101
circulatory failure 95
circumcision 133
clinical governance 138
clotrimazole 76
coarctation of the aorta 51
coeliac disease 33, 40, 42
  flat mucosa 40, *41*, 42
  guidance for parents 151
colonic inertia 148
Common Assessment Framework (CAF) 125
common cold 10, 13
communication 1
  interprofessional 124
  outpatient clinics 132
  social care 145
  three-year olds 5
community services 128–30, 132
compulsions 105
computer system 128
confusion, toddlers 4
congenital adrenal hyperplasia 56
congenital heart disease 51, *52*, 56
  rubella in pregnancy 67
coning 78
consciousness loss 96
  diabetic ketoacidosis 97
constipation 148
  typhoid fever 67
consultant paediatricians 128–9
contact allergy 69
convulsions 97, 132
  antihistamine poisoning 89
  febrile 14, 77–9
coryza 10
cough
  acute 10

asthma 21
  chickenpox 65
  measles 64, 65
  persistent 11
  pneumonia 11
  recurrent 21
  sudden onset 19
  vomiting in whooping cough 37
  whooping cough 11–12
cow's milk protein intolerance 40–41, 42, 97
coxalgia fugax 119
Coxsackie virus 62
crotamiton cream 75
crying, guidance for parents 151
cryotherapy 73
Cryptosporidium 36, 40
cyanosis 97
cycling 90–91
cystic fibrosis 11, 13, 41, 56
  guidance for parents 151
  neonatal screen 41
cystourethrography 46, *47*
cytomegalovirus (CMV) 147

data collection 125, **127, 139**
day centres 111
day-care 132–3
deaths 143
defecation, pain 148
dehydration
  gastroenteritis 35, 36, 37
  severely ill child 96
dependence 3, 5
depression
  maternal of toddlers 3
  postnatal 125
deprivation 56
dermatitis 71–2
dermatology 69–76
desmopressin 49
desquamation *62*, 63
detergents 150–51
developing countries
  gastroenteritis 36–7
  measles 65
developmental delay 5
  epilepsy 80
  HIV/AIDS 68
developmental disorders 108–9
  assessment process 109–10
  diagnosis 110
  education 111
  interventions/management 110
  parental reactions 110–11
  treatment 111
  voluntary sector 111
dexamethasone 18
diabetes mellitus 132
  guidance for parents 152
diabetic ketoacidosis 30, 97
diarrhoea 35–7
  chronic 39–42, 56
  HIV/AIDS 68
  measles 65
  plant ingestion 86
  typhoid fever 67
diazepam 77, 78, *78*, 97

diphtheria 14
disability 108
    guidance for parents 151–2
    outpatient services 131
    parental reactions 110–11
Disability Living Allowance 110
disobedience 106
disruptive behaviour 106
domestic violence 113
Down's syndrome 108
    guidance for parents 152
drowsiness 96
    stridor 97
drug rash 61
    measles 65
drugs 151
    asthma 24–6
    sleep problem treatment 7
ductus arteriosus, patent 51, *52*
dyslexia 113

ear examination 15
Early Bird parent programme 111
eating
    healthy 59
    toddlers 4
econazole 76
eczema
    guidance for parents 152
    herpeticum 70
    impetigo 71
    lick 72
    see also atopic eczema
education 112
    developmental disorders 111
    parental impact 114
Education Act (1993) 110
Education Act (1996) 130
educational assessment 112
emergencies 124
    services 134
emollients 70
emotional disorders
    abdominal pain 32, 33
    gait abnormality 121
    nocturnal enuresis 50
    school failure 113
    short stature 55
emotional tension, headache 84
encephalitis, measles 64–5
endoscopy 133
enuresis 132
    see also nocturnal enuresis
enuresis alarms 49
epiglottitis 97
    acute 19
epilepsy 80–82, 108
    differential diagnosis 81–2
    guidance for parents 152
    investigations 82
    management 82
    syndromes 80
Epstein–Barr virus (EBV) 67
equipment 2
erythema infectiosum 66–7
ethosuximide 81
Every Child Matters 125

evidence-based practice 125
executive functioning problems 113
exercise, increase 59

failure to thrive 132
    HIV/AIDS 68
famciclovir 70
family
    developmental disorder effects 110
    epilepsy 82
    healthy eating 59
    physical activity 59
    reaction to behaviour problems 5
    recurrent abdominal pain 32
    school failure 113–14
farm safety 92
fears 106
febrile convulsions 14, 77–9
    advice to parents **79**
    complex **79**
    emergency treatment 77–8
    information for parents 79
    prognosis 78, 79
    severely ill children 97
    treatment 78
feet, flat 117–18
femoral anteversion/retroversion, persistent 117
femoral epiphysis
    injury 121
    slipped upper 119
femoral head, Perthes' disease 119–20
femoral pulse 51, *52*
ferritin levels 149
fever 102–4
    detection 102
    duration 10
    investigations 102–3
    management 78, 102–3
    meningitis 37
    pneumonia 11
    pyelonephritis 44
    risk assessment 102, **103**
    roseola infantum 65
    scarlet fever 66
    tonsillitis 14
    typhoid fever 67
    see also febrile convulsions
fifth disease 66–7
fires 91–2
flat feet 117–18
food
    anaphylactic reaction 42
    asthma precipitation 24
    deficiency 55–6
    intolerance 42
food tolerance tests 133
foreign body 19–20
    inhaled 97
    leg pain 120
    vaginal 151
formula milk 150
fractures
    child abuse 142
    hospital admission 135
    minor leg 120
fungal infections 76
    napkin dermatitis 72

gait
    complex disturbance 121
    see also limp
gastric aspiration 96, 97
gastric dilatation 97
gastric lavage 87
gastroenteritis 31, 35–7, 42
    acute 96–7
    hospital admission 36, 135, 136–7
    intravenous fluids 135
general practice, organization 122
general practitioners
    home visits 123–4
    hospital admissions 135
    referrals 131
    services 122–5, **126, 127**
    see also primary care
genital warts 72
genitalia
    examination 142, 143
    testis torsion 30, 67
German measles 67
Giardia 40
gingivostomatitis, acute herpetic 147
glandular fever *see* infectious mononucleosis
glucose
    blood concentration 97
    blood test 95
glucose–electrolyte mixture 36
glue ear 16
glues 87
grief 110
griseofulvin 76
grommets 16, 17, 133
growth
    atypical patterns 55
    curve 56
    failure 53–6, 132
    familial patterns 54–5
    normal 39
growth charts 53, *54*, 56
growth hormone deficiency 56
gut malrotation 33

habits 105
    toddlers 4
haemangiomas 75
haemoglobin electrophoresis 149
haemoglobin S 149
haemoglobinopathies 149–50
Haemophilus influenzae 19
hair
    fungal infections 76
    pediculosis capitis 73, *74*
    pulling 105
hallucinations 81
    antihistamine poisoning 89
hand, foot and mouth disease 62
harm, significant 142
head injury
    child abuse 142
    migraine 84
head louse 73
headache
    diabetic ketoacidosis 97
    intracranial lesions 84–5
    meningitis 37

headache (*Contd.*)
  recurrent 83–5
  scarlet fever 66
  tension 83, 84
  typhoid fever 67
head-banging 105
health visitors 109, 125, 129–30
healthy eating 59
hearing loss 5, 16, 108, 132
  guidance for parents 151
hearing test 15, *16*
heart disease, congenital 51, *52*, 56
heart rate 95
Heimlich manoeuvre 19–20
Henoch–Schönlein purpura 30, 60, *61*
hepatitis
  infectious mononucleosis complication 67
  jaundice 150
  measles 65
hepatitis A virus 150
hernia
  inguinal 30
  repair 133
herpes simplex encephalitis **104**
herpes simplex virus (HSV)
  Kaposi's varicelliform eruption 70
  mouth 147
herpes zoster, vesicles 61–2
herpetic gingivostomatitis 147
hip
  congenital dislocation *120*
  irritable 119
history taking 1
  asthma 22
HIV/AIDS 68
home, accidents in 91–2
home nursing care teams 135
home visits 123–4
hookfoot 115
hospital admission 135
  abdominal pain 33
  appendicitis 135
  asthma 26–7, 135
  bronchiolitis 135
  child abuse 143
  febrile convulsions 77
  fractures 135
  gait disorders 121
  gastroenteritis 36, 135, 136–7
  indications 135
  infectious diseases 136–7
  inguinal hernia 30
  laryngotracheitis 18
  mothers 136
  non-accidental injury 135, 143
  planned 137
  pneumonia 11
  poisoning 87
  preparation 137
  procedure 135
  pyelonephritis 44
  reasons 135–6
  sickle cell disease 30
  typhoid fever 68
  whooping cough 12
hospital referral, growth failure 56
hospital-at-home services 124

household products 86–7
human herpesvirus 6/7 65
hydrocortisone 42, 69, 72
hypertension, renal scarring 43

ibuprofen 10, 14
  fever 104
idiopathic thrombocytopenic purpura 60
imaging
  abdominal radiography 33
  renal scan 133
  urinary tract infection 46, *47*
  see also chest radiograph
imidazoles 76
immune deficiency 11
immunization 124–5
  febrile convulsions 78
  schedule 125, 128
  typhoid fever 68
immunoglobulin G (IgG) subclasses 11
immunoglobulins, plasma levels 11, 13
impetigo 70, *71*
independence 3
Individual Education Plan (IEP) 110
infectious diseases 64–8, 136–7
  see also bacterial infections; fungal infections;
    named diseases; viral infections
infectious mononucleosis 14, 61, 67, 147
  chronic fatigue syndrome 106
inflammatory bowel disease 33
inguinal hernia 30
injury, limp 119–21
insect bites/stings 42, 60
insecurity 3
insulin, diabetic ketoacidosis 97
intellectual disability 112
  mental retardation with rubella 67
  school failure 113
interagency working 145
  collaboration 146
intestinal obstruction 29, 98
  gut malrotation 33
intracranial abscess 84, *85*
intracranial lesions 84–5
intracranial pressure, raised in meningitis 38
intravenous fluids 36, 38, 95
  diabetic ketoacidosis 97
  gastroenteritis 135
intussusception 29–30
invalidity, guidance for parents 152
ipratropium bromide 27
iron
  poisoning 88–9
  supplementation 149
iron deficiency anaemia 148–9, 150
irritable bowel syndrome (IBS) 33
irritable hip 119
itching, nocturnal 69, 70

jaundice 150
jejunal biopsy 40, 42
joint laxity 118
joint swelling, Henoch–Schönlein purpura 30
juvenile arthritis 119

kaposi's varicelliform eruption 70
Kawasaki disease **104**

kerion *76*
ketoacidosis, diabetic 30
knee
  deformity 117
  hyperextension 118
  pain 120
knock knees 117
Koebner phenomenon 72
Koplik spots 61, 64

labyrinthitis, acute 81–2
lactase deficiency 40, *41*
lamotrigine 81
language
  development delay 5, 113
  see also speech
laryngitis 97
  acute 18–19
laryngotracheitis, acute 18–19
learning difficulties 112, 113
  guidance for parents 152
leg
  inequality 120–21
  limp 119–21
  minor orthopaedic problems 115–18
  pain 119–20
leukaemia 119, 137, 147
leukotriene receptor antagonists 25, 27
lick eczema 72
life support 100–101
limp 119–21
  pain 119–20
lindane 75
liquid nitrogen 73
liver
  congestive cardiac failure 97
  paracetamol poisoning 88
local education authorities 111, 112
Local Safeguarding Children Boards (LSCBs) 124
louse infestation *see* pediculosis
lumbar puncture 78
lung disease, cystic fibrosis 41
lymph node biopsy 147
lymphadenopathy, suboccipital 60
lymphoma 147

macules 60, *61*
maculopapular rash 61, *62,* 64, 66, 67
malabsorption 55–6
  coeliac disease 42
malathion 73
malnutrition 55–6
malrotation of the gut 33
Mantoux test 11, 13
mastoiditis 15
maturation, delayed 48, 55
measles 61, *62,* 64–5
medial tibial torsion 115–16
medical staff, strains 136
memory problems 113
meningitis 37–8, 78, **104**
  rash 37, 98, *99*
meningococcal disease **104**
  rash 60
mental health problems 112, 113
  see also anxiety; depression
mental retardation, rubella in pregnancy 67

metatarsus varus/adductus 115, *116*
metered dose inhalers 25, 27
methyl salicylate 87
miconazole 76
Microsporum canis 76
micturition cystogram 133
midazolam 77, 78, 97
migraine 83–4
misunderstanding 4
molluscum contagiosum 72, 73
Monilia 150
Monospot screening test 147
mothers
    hospital admissions 136
    terrible twos 3–4
mouth breathing 17
Movicol 148
multidisciplinary teams 109, 110
mumps 67
mupirocin 71
muscular dystrophy 121
Mycobacterium tuberculosis
        (tuberculosis) 12
myelomeningocele 108
myoclonic epilepsy 81
myringotomy 16

nail-biting 105
napkin dermatitis 71–2
nasal drops 10
nebulizer 13, 25
neglect 56
neonatal follow-up clinics 132
neurodevelopmental problems 113, 132
newborn infants 137
nightmares 6–7
nits 73, *74*
nocturnal enuresis 48–50
    buzzer treatment 49
non-accidental injury 132, 141–3
    hospital admission 135, 143
    photographs 142, 143
non-poisons 86–7
nurseries, specialist 111
nurses
    home nursing care team 135
    paediatric wards 136
    school 130
    specialist teams 130
    strains 136
    triage 134
nystatin 72

obesity 57, *58,* 59
    early detection 57
    management 57, 59
    prevention 57
    support 59
onychomycosis 76
opiates 87
oral rehydrating fluids 36, 37
orchitis 30, 67
orthopaedic problems
    limp 119–21
    minor 115–18
osteochondrosis 120
osteomyelitis **104,** 119

otitis media 10
    acute 13, 14–15
    hearing loss 108
    measles complication 64
    secretory 15–17
out-of-hours calls 123–4
outpatient clinics 131–2
    appointment systems 132
out-toeing 117
oxygen therapy 18, 94, 95
    anaphylaxis 42
    asthma 26

paediatric emergencies 124
paediatricians, community child
        health 128–9
pain
    defecation 148
    leg 119–20
    see also abdominal pain
paints 87
papules 60, *61*
paracetamol 10, 14, 78, 84
    fever 104
    herpetic gingivostomatitis 147
    poisoning 88
paraffin, poisoning 89
parental illness 113
parental separation 112, 113
parents
    advice on febrile convulsions **79**
    assessment 1
    attitudes to school 112
    benign systolic murmurs 52
    counseling for HIV/AIDS 68
    developmental delay identification 109
    educational impact 114
    epilepsy 82
    fever management 104
    guidance 151–2
    inconsistency 4
    information 151–2
        febrile convulsions 79
        urinary tract infection **45**
    reaction to developmental disorders 110–11
    recurrent abdominal pain management 32,
        33–4
    sleep problem management 7, **8,** 9
    support groups 111
    talking about social care concerns 145
    terrible twos 3–4
paroxysmal supraventricular tachycardia 97
partial seizures 81
parvovirus B19 66, 67
patellae, squinting 117
patent ductus arteriosus 51, *52*
peak flow rate 22
pediculosis
    capitis 73, *74*
    impetigo 71
periodic syndrome 30–31
peritonsillar abscess 14
permethrin 73, 75
persistent femoral anteversion/retroversion 117
personal child health record 128
Perthes' disease 119–20
pesticides 87

pharyngitis 14
phenothiazines, poisoning 88
phenothrin 73
physical activity 59
physical difficulties, school failure 112
physical disability 109
physical examination 2
    appendicitis 29
physiotherapy, chest 12
pityriasis alba 71
pizotifen 84
plants, non-poisonous 86
play 1, 2
    in hospital 136
playground equipment, accidents 92
playgroups, specialist 111
pneumonia *98,* **104**
    HIV/AIDS 68
    lobar 11
    measles 65
    respiratory rate 97
    segmental 11
poisoning 86–9
poliomyelitis 121
polyethylene glycol (PEG) 148
postnatal depression 125
postviral syndrome 67, 106–7
Poxviridae 73
prednisolone 26, 75
pregnancy
    HIV treatment 68
    parvovirus infection 67
    rubella 67
preterm infants 137
preventive care 124–5
primary care 122–5, **126, 127**
    audit 138–40
    child health surveillance 125, 128, **129**
    data collection 125, **127**
    emergency department 134
    evidence-based practice 125
    home visits 123–4
    medical equipment 122–3
    organization 122
    out-of-hours calls 123–4
    preventive 124–5
    referrals 124
    service provision 124, 128
primary health care team
        (PHCT) 124
promethazine 37, 66
propranolol 84
protection *see* child protection
pruritus
    atopic eczema 69
    scabies 75
psoriasis 63
psychiatric disorders
    abdominal pain 34
    nocturnal enuresis 50
puberty
    acceleration 55
    early 57
pulmonary stenosis 51
pulse rate 95
purpura 60
pyelonephritis 44

quality of care 138
questioning the child 1–2
quinsy 14

rash 60–61, *62*, 63
    anaphylaxis 42
    chickenpox 61, *62*, 65, 66
    Henoch–Schönlein purpura 30
    infectious mononucleosis 67
    maculopapular 61, *62*, 64, 66, 67
    measles 61, *62*, 64, 65
    meningitis 37, 98, 99
    meningococcal disease 60
    rubella 67
    scarlet fever 66
    severely ill children 98, *99*
rat bait 87
rectal polyp 148
referral 124
    child abuse 142
    child protection 146
    Children's Social Care 5
    growth failure 56
    outpatient services 131
    social care 144, 145
    welfare concerns 144
rehydration 96
renal failure 43
renal scan 133
renal scarring 43, 46, *47*
resentment 4
respiratory rate 94
    raised 97, *98*
respiratory syncytial virus 11, 12, 13
respiratory tract infection 10–13
    migraine 84
    recurrent 13, 132
respite care 110
rickets 116, 150
road accidents 90–91
roseola 60, 65
rotavirus 35–6, 40
rubella 60, 67

salbutamol 26, 37
    anaphylaxis 42
    whooping cough 12
salicylates 87
salicylic acid 73
Salmonella 36
Salmonella typhi 67
Sarcoptes scabiei 73, *74*
scabies 73, *74*, 75
    impetigo 71
scalds, stridor 19
scales, weighing 122, *123*
scarlet fever 66
school failure 112–14
    child factors 112–13
    emotional difficulties 113
    family factors 113–14
    intellectual disability 113
    learning difficulties 113
    mental health problems 112, 113
    neurodevelopmental
        problems 113
    physical difficulties 112

school factors 114
    sensory difficulties 112
school health service 130
school nurses 130
school/school factors
    abdominal pain 33
    absence 112
    children's attitudes 112
    migraine 83, 84
    parent attitudes 112
    problems 112
    return after chronic fatigue
        syndrome 106–7
seborrhoeic dermatitis 71
secondary care, service provision 128
security 3
seizures
    partial 81
    types 80
    see also epilepsy
senna 148
sensory difficulties, school failure 112
separation 3, 5
septic arthritis **104**, 119
services
    ambulatory paediatrics 134–5
    community 128–30
    emergency department 134
    primary care 122–5, **126, 127**
    social care 144–6
    see also child health services
severely ill children 94–8, *99*
    abdominal tenderness 98
    convulsions 97
    diabetic ketoacidosis 97
    gastroenteritis 96–7
    guidance for parents 151–2
    hospital admission 135
    identification **103**
    immediate management 94–5
    rash 98, *99*
    respiratory rate increase 97, *98*
    urgent investigations 96
sexual abuse 143
Shigella 36
short stature, familial 55
sickle cell disease 30, *31*, 66, 149, 150
sinusitis, migraine 84
skewfoot 115
skin conditions 69–76
slapped cheek syndrome 66
sleep, normal patterns 6
sleep apnoea 17
sleep problems 6–7, **8**, 9
    behaviour modification 7
    drug treatment 7
    early waking 9
    getting to sleep 7
    history 6–7, **8**
    toddlers 4
slipped upper femoral epiphysis 119
smoke detectors 91, *92*
snoring 17
social care 144–6
    assessment 146
    eligibility criteria 145
    information sharing 145

referral 144, 145
    thresholds 145
social class, accidents 90
social problems 56
social services 144
social workers, response to concerns 145–6
sodium valproate 80, 81
soiling, overflow 148
sore throat 10, 14
    recurrent 17
spacer device 13, 25, 27
special care baby units 132, 137
special educational needs 111, 130
special needs, children with 108–11
special needs coordinator (SENCO) 111
specialist nurse teams 130
speech 3
    problems 5
    see also language
spinal dysraphism 120, 121
spinal lesion 48
spinal tumours 121
spleen, ruptured 30
squinting patellae 117
Standard Assessment Tests (SATs) 112, 114
Staphylococcus aureus 19, 69–70
star chart 48–9
steam inhalation 18
steatorrhoea, cystic fibrosis 41
steroids
    inhaled 13, 25, 26
    oral 26, 27
    topical 69, 70
streptococci, haemolytic 14, 17, 66
stress
    migraine 83
    school failure 114
stridor 18–20
    severely ill children 97
subdural haemorrhage 84
suboccipital lymphadenopathy 60
sucrose solution 36
sudden infant death syndrome (SIDS) 125, 143
supraventricular tachycardia, paroxysmal 97
surgery, day-care 133
surgical shock 30
sweat test 11, 13, 40, 41, 56
    day-care unit 133
sweets 2
swimming pools 92
syncope 81
synovitis, transient 119
systolic murmurs 51–2, 132
    benign origin 52

talking 1–2
    with children 145
teachers 114
temper tantrum 3, 4
temperament 4
temperature taking 102
terbinafine 76
terbutaline 26
    anaphylaxis 42
testis, torsion 30, 67
thalassaemia 149–50
thrombocytopenic purpura 60

thumb-sucking 105
tibia
    physiological bowing 115–16
    vara 116
tics 105
tinea capitis/cruris/pedis 76
toddlers 3–5
toilet training 5
tonic–clonic epilepsy 80, 81
tonsillectomy, indications 17
tonsillitis 13, 14
    scarlet fever 66
torsion of testis 30, 67
toxoplasma 147
toys 1, 2, 151, *152*
    sleep disturbance 7, 9
trauma
    abdominal pain 30
    femoral epiphysis 121
    head injury 84, 142
    limp 119–21
    sleep disturbance 7
tretinoin 73
triage nurse 134
Trichomonas 150
Trichophyton mentagrophytes 76
Trichophyton tonsurans 76
tricyclic antidepressants 50
trypsin, blood immunoreactive level 41
tuberculosis 11, 12–13, 119
tumours 119
Turner's syndrome 56
turpentine, poisoning 89
tympanic membrane 15, 16
tympanogram *16*
typhoid fever 67–8

ultrasound examination
    abdomen 33
    urinary tract infection 46, *47*

understanding 3
urinary tract infection 30, 43–7, **104**
    audit *140*
    clinical features 43
    diagnostic criteria 44
    enuresis 48
    imaging 46, *47*
    information for parents **45**
    prophylaxis 47
    specimen transport 44
    urine collection 44
urine
    examination 30, 33
    microscopy 44
    specimen transport 44
urticaria, papular 60

valaciclovir 70
vascular anomalies 75, 84
ventilation 42
    bag and mask 95
ventricular septal defect 51, 52
verrucae 72, *73*, 120
vertigo 82
vesicles 61–2
vesicoureteric reflux 43, 46, *47*
    prophylaxis 47
viral infections
    cervical lymphadenopathy 147
    laryngotracheitis 19
    otitis media 14–15
    secondary 69
    tonsillitis 14
    vertigo 82
    see also named infections
visual defects 108
    guidance for parents 151
vitamin D 150
voluntary sector, developmental disorders 111
volvulus 33

vomiting 35–8
    abdominal pain 31, 32
    anaphylaxis 42
    gastroenteritis 35–7
    meningitis 37–8
    plant ingestion 86
    salicylate poisoning 87
    whooping cough 37
vulnerable children 145
vulvovaginitis 150–51

warfarin 87
warts 72–3
wasting 53–4, 56
weedkillers 87
weight gain, poor 40
welfare concerns, referral 144
wheals *62*, 63
wheezing 11
    asthma 21
Whitfield's ointment 76
whooping cough 11–12, 37
Wood's lamp 76
Working Together to Safeguard Children (DoH
    1999, rev 2006) 141

zinc ointment BP 72